The Encyclopedia of Alternative Health Care brings you effective therapies from all over the globe—all of which are in use in the United States today. In this practical guide, you'll discover indispensable information on options such as:

- *Aromatherapy:* Essental oils extracted from plants are the basis of this treatment. Modern aromatherapy, developed in France, is used to treat poor circulation, obesity, rheumatism, sinusitis, depression, and stress . . .
- *Past Life Therapy:* Eastern beliefs in reincarnation and Western psychology combine in this therapy. Problems that respond particularly well to past life therapy include: phobias, compulsions, asthma, and chronic back pain . . .
- *Iridology:* Traditionally believed to have originated in ancient Greece, iridology is the study of how the eye reveals health problems. Iridologists study the eyes for indications of nutritional deficiencies, nervous disorders, congested organs, and glandular problems . . .
- *Homeopathy:* Originating in Germany, homeopathy quickly became popular in nineteenth-century Europe and America and is used by the British royal family today. Homepathic remedies are particularly effective for chronic problems (such as ulcers and high blood pressure), mild deficiencies (such as anemia), allergies (especially hay fever and food allergies), and prevention of problems such as miscarriages and bruising . . .
- *And much more in . . . THE ENCYCLOPEDIA OF ALTERNATIVE HEALTH CARE*

The
ENCYCLOPEDIA
of ALTERNATIVE
HEALTH CARE

Kristin Gottschalk Olsen

Produced by The Philip Lief Group, Inc.

POCKET BOOKS

New York   London   Toronto   Sydney   Tokyo   Singapore

This book is a reference book which is intended to supplement, not replace, the advice of a trained health professional. The opinions expressed herein are not necessarily those of, nor endorsed by, the publisher. If you know or suspect you have a health problem, you should consult a trained health professional.

An *Original* Publication of POCKET BOOKS

 POCKET BOOKS, a division of Simon & Schuster Inc.
1230 Avenue of the Americas, New York, NY 10020

Copyright © 1989 by Kristin L. Olsen
Cover art copyright © 1990 Carol Gillot

Produced by The Philip Lief Group, Inc.

ISBN: 0-671-73552-7

First Pocket Books trade paperback printing January 1990

10 9 8 7 6 5 4 3 2

POCKET and colophon are registered trademarks
of Simon & Schuster Inc.

Printed in the U.S.A.

This book is dedicated to all my sisters . . .

Especially
Lt. Jennie C. Olsen, R.N.
and
Mari Siv Kvaale
Who, in their very different worlds and unique ways,
are true healers

and
Berit

Acknowledgments

Many practitioners have shared with me their knowledge, insights, skills, enthuiasm, and gifts. As professionals, as friends, as interviewees, they have taught me about their particular healing modalities, about healing as a process, and about myself as a human being. A number of practitioners provided information and/or reviewed and made suggestions for selected chapters.

Thanks to the caring people for sharing ideas and feelings, laughs, and caring attention from the heart: Michael Reed Gach, Howard Harrison, Rose Adams Kelly, Kurt Schnaubelt, Dev Priya and Ashwin Hansen, Lynn Rabinov Vespe, Margaret Buck, Leslie Kaslof, Richie A. Heckler, Mitchell Corwin, William Meeker, Barney Coyle, Nancy Gardner, Frank Wildman, Greg Schelkun, Savita, Candace Schoonover, Holly Holmes, Jeff Bruno, Paul Reinhertz, Judith McKinnon, Carol Lourie, Cheryl Whitaker, Hazel Denning, Ray Castellino, Michael O'Leary, Audrey L. Seymour, Mary Kay Wright-Malear, Cynthia Payne Cramer, Sue Ann Dunford, Gail Stewart, Ron Valle, Robert Shubow, David Zimmerman and Jean North.

So many of the people mentioned above mirror for me how deeply we can integrate the holistic philosophy into our lives, our work, our relationships, and our health.

I also want to thank Philip Lief who made this project possible, Nancy Kalish who midwifed with TLC both the author and the manuscript, Scott Corngold for his insightful blue pencil, Claire Zion for her vision as editor, and Carol Gillot for the exquisite cover art.

Next, I want to acknowledge the many special people I met at John F. Kennedy University during my years in its Holistic Health Education program. JFKU, particularly its Graduate School for the Study of Human Consciousness, attracts an unusual kind of student. Adult learners from all over the world pass through its process-oriented programs, transforming their lives as well as their careers. Both the people and the place were central to my transformation process, which has culminated in my new role as a health educator and communicator. Thanks also goes to the University's Communications Office and its Robert M. Fisher Library for affectionate support and indulgence.

My deep gratitude goes to Dr. Frank Shallenberger, who not only wrote the superb foreword to this volume but also bore the brunt of my learning curve as a participating health client. His patience in the face of my initial hostility, his insights and openness, as well as his talents as a physician, showed me the possibilities of enlightened Western medicine.

I also wish to acknowledge Willis Harmon and Brendan O'Regan at the Institute of Noetic Sciences for planting the initial seeds of my interest in health research and writing; to mention Whole Life Expo 1988 for an opportunity to tour the sometimes hard-sell end of this new health industry; and thank my support group—Sue Ann Dunford, Carolyn Erskine, Ruby Okasaki, and Laurie Trujillo. Both as individuals and as a group they embody the highest good of holism, friendship, and actualized lifelong learning.

Finally, love and thanks to my Lafayette extended family: Bill Clark, who kept me light; Diana C. Wood, who revived my fatiguing arms and shoulders after long hours at the computer; and Tracy Woodruff for helping me take timely breaks from the writing process for walks, talks, and gardening. And my deepest appreciation to Michael Anne Conley who not only plugged me into this project, but also kept the juices running with her insights, encouragement, and occasional tussles with prepositions and pronouns. Great friends are the best medicine!

Namasté,
Kristin Gottschalk Olsen
Orinda, California
May 4, 1989

Contents

SECTION 1

A NEW HEALTH CARE LIFESTYLE

SECTION 2

THE HEALING ARTS

xii *Contents*

Preface

Health care in America has reached an exciting crossroad. The number of healing arts, practitioners, and people interested in what some call "alternative medicine" is growing to a critical mass, fueling a new holistic health care industry. Frustrated health consumers are aggressively seeking information and new choices for their health care. Many are making personal peace between orthodox medicine ("allopathic medicine") and alternative practices, forging their own complementary medicine out of resources from both markets. *Encyclopedia of Alternative Health Care* is designed as an aid for raising your consciousness about this new complementary approach.

My intent in writing this book is to demystify holistic health. This book is a tool for motivated health care consumers to use to inform themselves about the possibilities of the new complementary medicine. People interested in holistic health need perspective and a place to start looking for these resources. *Encyclopedia of Alternative Health Care* is a map, an outline of a territory about to be settled with a massive new wave of immigrants. I have also highlighted skills that are useful when participating in a healing partnership, since participation is part of the holistic healing process. Use this volume as a resource to begin your own exploration of the holistic health field.

Advances in medical technology have given us the means to do what no other medicinal system has done before in the way of saving lives. However, the focus on technological medicine has also starved the typical patient of the *human* elements of healing. The new popularity of holistic healing arts seems to be an attempt to recapture that human dimension. We are coming full circle, back to the conventional wisdom of what the idea of the old family doctor represents: someone who takes the time to provide a human touch and emotional contact. All kinds of healers—from physicians to counselors to bodyworkers—are recognizing the importance of treating the whole person and not just the disease.

More and more people are attending classes to learn such self-help routines as relaxation techniques, yoga, massage, special nutritional practices, and a variety of bodywork techniques. Others read through resource guides like the San Francisco Bay Area's *Commonground* for practitioners and health centers. Many who are helped by a particular healing art or practitioner end up training in that healing modality, swelling the ranks of amateur and professional holistic health practitioners.

This holistic health movement represents a third generation of professionals. Like the settlers who carved out farms and ranches or built the towns of the Old West, the current generation of healing arts professionals is creating a new holistic health care industry. These health care practitioners are not only putting down roots, but they're also staking their claims in the new health care market. Those at the leading edges of the holistic industry are using conferences, summit meetings, the media, courts, and legislatures to promote, define, standardize, and license their particular practices. Professional organizations are networking and politicking to discern and distinguish individual methodologies, professional languages, and marketplaces. The creators of healing modalities are registering their trademark names and logos. Teachers and practitioners are organizing into guilds, institutes, or other nonprofit entities. Organizations are incorporating and, along with a growing number of for-profit businesses, providing a wide range of services and products. Holistic health seems to have come of age.

Health is a living process, a dynamic series of events and plateaus, turns and stops along the spiral toward wellness or illness. Health is very personal. It has to be because it is about our bodies—the beings we are 24 hours a day, 365 days a year, for our entire lives. We can never get away from our health, even when we sleep. It is not just a part of us—it *is* us.

As a living process, health is constantly changing. How active you want to be in creating and directing both the process and direction of that change is up to you. We *can* change ourselves, but it takes time, motivation, help, and lots of self-love. Support from friends and access to resources make the process run more easily.

The ideas, approaches, and healing arts profiles I present in this book were gathered on my journey from a passive medical patient to a responsible health client. They are only a beginning.

A proverb says you can give a man a fish and feed him for a day. But teach that man to fish and you feed him for a lifetime. Hopefully, this book will be a fishing pole for lifelong learning about yourself and the health care resources that work for you.

Information empowers individuals to take more responsibility for their health care. Empowered health care consumers have a sense of themselves and what they want and need. They are open and inquisitive, as well as assertive and critical. They demand competence from practitioners, are aware of the effects of any health care session, treatment, or consultation, and have a sense of what works or doesn't work for them.

Getting to that point is hard, though, because our culture encourages us to shrug off self-awareness and the responsibility for our health. Many of us grow up learning that sickness is something that happens *to* us and that getting well is up to someone or something else—usually doctors or drugs.

I used to be one of those helpless people. I was getting sicker and more angry that "the doctors" couldn't find what was really wrong with me. It took some painful and scary experiences to wake me up to the fact that I *could* and *would* have to do something about my own state of health.

The changes I had to make in myself and my lifestyle offered a number of lessons and pushed me through several roles. I went from being an unconscious "victim" of illness and a passive medical patient to an antimedication zealot after the panic of an allergic reaction to overprescribed penicillin.

In an effort to avoid all doctors, I became a holistic health explorer, making myself my own guinea pig as I experimented with various home remedies and consulted alternative healing arts professionals. Eventually, the "bad" experiences I had at the hands of both conventional physicians and supposedly holistic practitioners galvanized me into becoming an educated and responsible consumer of both kinds of health care.

My explorations taught me the benefits of using a wider choice of healing modalities and of taking a participatory role in my own health care. It also showed me the dangers of approaching health care with prejudicial blinders restricting my point of view. I learned new ways to approach eating and nutrition, discovered bodywork's healing effects on both my mind and body, and gained insight into some of my behavior patterns and relationships through past life and other psychotherapies. Most important, I developed a holistic view and appreciation of myself as a person.

However, at one point, I began to feel very sick. My alternative solutions helped only sometimes. I resisted going back to medical doctors because the memory of their arrogance and insensitivity was still fresh. It took a serious crisis to scare me enough to seek out one. When I did, Dr. Frank Shallenberger not only listened with patience but gave me the overview, scientific perspective, and technical understanding of disease process and physiology that I lacked. He also showed me that some doctors were willing and capable of participating in a healing partnership.

Encyclopedia of Alternative Health Care is not meant to be used as a source of medical advice, nor for the diagnosis or treatment of disease. I *do* mean to encourage you to evaluate any ideas presented to you—in my book, or by any practitioner, doctor, or authority figure. And I *do* mean to encourage you to participate in your own healing process by finding the approaches or methods that give you meaning as well as results.

I continue to live my own health spiral, moving from one plateau to another, continually returning to old issues or goals, but at a new level of experience or understanding. This book represents just the early phases of my personal health odyssey. I expect to continue exploring health care options for as long as I live. There are so many more choices and resources still in development—and yet to be created—that may help me. The fun is as much in the discovery as in the accomplishment or completion of a goal. And, I now know that I have a wide circle of resources for support—friends and professionals with whom I have created healing relationships and helping partnerships.

Foreword

Not long ago, I obtained a copy of Hippocrates' writings. Until then, the only thing I knew about Hippocrates was that he practiced medicine more than 2,000 years ago and that he wrote the Oath of Ethics that all medical students take upon graduation. As I read his words, I was surprised to realize that much of what he was teaching then is relevant to the current state of health care in the United States. He wrote about healing patients with food as opposed to drugs. He emphasized knowing the patient's personality type, diet, and occupation as necessary determinants of the course of therapy given. He even went so far as to spend a lot of time detailing how food allergies or intolerances can play a large role in the genesis of disease.

I soon began to wonder how Hippocrates would be appreciated if he were practicing his art today. He would undoubtedly be very busy, with people coming from all parts to see him. Most of those people would probably be patients for whom the conventional approach to health care—consisting of medication, radiation, and surgery—had failed, caused intolerable side effects, or been unacceptable in some other way.

Soon, as his reputation spread, patients would see him for problems even before they consulted their regular medical doctors. At this point, knowing the medical community, most doctors would fall into one of three groups. One group, having heard of the wonderful success that Hippocrates was having with his different modalities, would want to learn more about what he was doing and investigate his methods closely. Another group would immediately label him a charlatan or a quack without bothering to investigate seriously what he was doing at all. They would simply insist that since his work was "unproven," "nonscientific," and "not generally accepted as normal for the medical community," it couldn't have much merit. Case closed. These doctors would be intent on saving gullible patients from being bilked by the old Greek and would start a vigilance committee against what they determined was health care fraud. The third group would generally not be too interested in Hippocrates one way or the other, and would take whatever course was the safest.

Eventually, because of the great controversy between the believers and the nonbelievers, misinformation and false accusations would flourish. After hearing the experts continually contradicting each other, people would be increasingly confused as to what to do for their health care problems. Many doctors would themselves be confused, not so sure anymore that conventional medicine was indeed the only valid way to create healing. To make matters worse, in the middle of all this would remain the ever-present subset of unscrupulous, self-labeled "health care practitioners" of various sorts who are poorly trained, uncertified, and who pose a threat to anyone entrusting their health care to them.

Such a stage would actually be very close to what we are experiencing today. Not infrequently, one of my patients will come to me and say that he has a relative who is seeing an acupuncturist or homeopath or "some doctor who is treating him with crystals." The patient will then quite naturally ask my opinion regarding this mode of therapy, about which I am more than likely quite ignorant. Usually I will ask him to check on the practitioner's education, training, certification, and reputation. I have always thought that well-educated, well-trained, certified professionals with a good reputation for producing results are probably going to keep on producing good results. I will also usually ask if the practitioner in question feels that his approach is the only valid approach. Usually, dogmatic types who are sure they have all the answers don't have many good ones.

Then comes another situation, the one in which I am working with a patient and not really helping her very much or maybe not at all. I start to wonder, if I can't, who can? Maybe she needs a whole new approach, but to whom do I refer her?

Finally, there is a third kind of situation, in which a patient comes to me for treatment at the same time she is receiving an "alternative" type of care from another practitioner. Is what I do going to complement or interfere with what is already being done?

Well, having experienced each of these scenarios many times over my 15 years of medical practice, I have to come around to developing a method of critiquing health and medical care. So now I ask six questions:

1) Is the therapy safe?
2) Does it have theoretical plausibility?
3) Is it relatively inexpensive?
4) Has it been around for more than a few years?
5) Has it been effective?
6) Is there no other therapy that meets all these criteria better?

If all these questions can be answered in the affirmative, then it seems likely that my patient might be on to something. Now, not wanting to be unfair, the first health care practice I started with was my own profession. I had been trained to practice conventional or "modern" medicine—so how did that stack up against these criteria?

As it turns out, the answer is "not so good." Conventional therapy isn't very safe. In fact, 30 percent of all office visits and 85 percent of all in-hospital complications are due to side effects from surgery and pharmaceuticals. As far as theory goes, we really don't have a very good idea of what most drugs do, and it just doesn't make a lot of sense to be putting foreign molecules we know so little about into our system. I remember Hippocrates admonishing "leave your chemicals in the chemist's pot if you can't cure your patient with foods."

Is it inexpensive? The answer is no. In fact, conventional medicine is 100 or 1,000 times more expensive than many other modalities. Has it been around more than a few years? Probably not. The general thrust of conventional medicine has been to use drugs that are relatively new. In fact, few doctors prescribe medications that have been in use more than 20 years. Conventional medicine does well at symptom alleviation and emergency trauma care, but in terms of problem-solving and disease prevention it is seriously lacking.

Lastly, are there any other kinds of treatments that meet these criteria better? I would hope so, but how does one go about finding that out in an intelligent and responsible way? It seems that this last question is the most important one of all. It is this basic issue, with all of its related spin-offs, that is addressed in this valuable and timely work. Kristin Gottschalk Olsen has not written just another "look over here, I found the answer" book, but a discourse designed to help you find your own special answer.

Hippocrates said, "It's more important to know what kind

of patient has a disease than what kind of disease a patient has.''
So your answer to health care is frequently going to need to take
into consideration more about your own uniqueness than about
the characteristics of your medical condition. As you read
through the pages of this book, I think you'll be able to see how
this all translates into an opportunity to take control of your
health, rather than leave it in the hands of fate or whim.

Frank A. Shallenberger, M.D.
Walnut Creek, California

How to Use This Book

Encyclopedia of Alternative Health Care is written as a guidebook for exploring holistic health care and complementary medicines. It is a tool to support changes for a healthier lifestyle.

The first section, "A New Health Care Lifestyle," provides some context for many new/old ideas of the holistic health movement. In "Just What Is Holistic Health?" I highlight basic concepts and explain some jargon used by people in the field. "Taking Charge" and "A New Generation of Practitioners" can help you prepare yourself for the process of taking more responsibility for your own health and finding help in doing it. The chapter "Participating in A Health Care Relationship" explains the role you and your health care professional play at each stage of a healing partnership.

"The Healing Spiral" helps you identify possible starting points for launching your explorations into a new health style, and tells about various different approaches, techniques, points of view, and experiences available in this burgeoning field of healing arts.

The second section, "The Healing Arts," profiles 33 major types of holistic practices. I chose the classics, the ones that have set the direction of the new health care, and I have often included discussion of derivative, complementary, or related healing arts. These are by no means all that are available to you as a consumer. There are many more types of health care practices to investigate. However, for the new explorer, the examples profiled are good places to start.

Many people start out looking for the one right healing art to fix a specific problem or complaint. However, what works for you today may change next year or with the next health problem. You can come back to the profiles again and again. Each time you might see something different, depending on how you feel or what you are seeking.

"The Healing Arts" profiles are listed alphabetically. For

each one or group, I start by giving an overview or a definition. Next, I include a brief history to give you an idea of the art's development into its present form.

In the third part of each profile, I talk about how the healing art works. To capture its character, I tend to use the same words the creators and practitioners of each form use themselves to describe their work. But I purposely observed and interviewed the students, not the creators of the healing arts, to provide some perspective. In many cases, I offer some physiology or examples to give an idea of how these techniques act on structure, functioning, and feelings.

Also included in each profile is something about the experience of the healing art, either describing a session or some effects of the technique. To gain some experience of each approach I have observed or taken sessions, classes, or trainings in almost all of the healing arts described.

Next I talk about how these healing arts are used. Some arts you can learn for yourself or use as a home remedy. Others are only administered by a practitioner or doctor, and address specific health problems.

I'm not necessarily making recommendations, but rather I offer a profile of effects as reported by the literature, practitioners, and clients. I have also provided warnings and cautions, where appropriate. One caution goes for all these profiles: Whether or not an approach has helped others, if you are under treatment or have a serious condition, consult your primary care provider before signing up for a specific new healing modality.

Finally, access to further investigation is provided at the end of each profile chapter. The addresses and book lists are tools for deeper exploration and information gathering.

I suggest you read the "Healing Spiral" chapter to get a feel for the different kinds of healing arts. Then read the profiles for those that appeal to you. Pay particular attention to how each one works and the experience of using it, not just to the possible benefits. After all, it can be an entirely new way for you to approach a health concern. Does it sound like something you would like and respond to if you tried it? Does it feel right for you?

Remember, building a healthy lifestyle is a daily experience. You may lose your motivation to complete a course of treatment or a health plan if you are in too much pain or if the approach is too disciplined or time-consuming. Think about what fits your lifestyle and level of commitment.

Remember, too, that this is just a beginning, an initial guide-book for you to use to explore new choices for a healthy lifestyle. I can't recommend any one of these for everybody. Each one works for some—but not all—people. Only you can decide what to try, what works and doesn't work to help you achieve your goals.

Your motivation, the relationship you create with the practi-tioner, your realistic expectations, and your past health history are as important as the actual healing techniques in making the experience valuable and determining the outcome. Go for it!

A New
Health Care
Lifestyle

Just What Is Holistic Health?

◇ **H**ealth care is in the middle of what the consciousness or "New Age" movement likes to call a "paradigm shift."
A paradigm is a set of beliefs, a point of view about the world. A
paradigm shift occurs when enough things happen to shake up
current thinking and thus, practices, on a grand scale.

At one time, people thought the world was flat and the sun
revolved around the earth. In that paradigm, the Earth was the
center of the universe. A whole series of rules, myths, facts,
religious beliefs, and nautical practices were based on these
"truths." You could sail off the end of the ocean if you went too
far west from Europe, for example. Pioneering sailors like Columbus and Magellan, whose explorations proved that the earth was
round, precipitated a major paradigm shift.

The "new age" philosophy, a marriage of Eastern and Western approaches and holism, a systemic awareness of the interrelatedness of all things, is beginning to shake up the current world
view. The shift has effects not only in world politics, but also in
the fields of mental and physical health.

Psychology is one science developing philosophies and techniques that encompass this shifting paradigm. Classical psychoanalysis now shares the mental health field with behavioral,
humanistic, and transpersonal psychologies. Each one approaches human emotions and behavior from different points of
view.

Transpersonal psychology incorporates the spiritual aspect,
combining Eastern philosophy with Western psychological techniques. In addition, with Freud's statement "anatomy is destiny"

3

coming full circle, a new somatic (body-oriented) psychology reemphasizes the importance of body awareness and influence on the psychoemotional experience.

By its very nature, holism is bringing health, psychology, and spirituality together into a "wholeness," or holistic approach to health care. This wholeness is slowly evolving into something more than just a marriage of different parts. It is becoming an entirely new attitude about the human experience of health.

The term *holistic* has come to mean different things to different people. Many products in the grocery store are called *natural*. However, when you read the label you find out that "natural" can mean the product contains no preservatives, but is full of sugars like corn syrup. Whereas other products labeled "natural" use unprocessed, whole grain ingredients and no sugars.

So too with professionals and practices labeled "holistic." Holistic can mean an approach different from orthodox medicine, a composite of many different techniques, or an awareness and respect for the person as a complex, multidimensional organism affected on all levels by that particular technique.

While I value a truly holistic attitude and think that it makes a difference in the experience of any healing art, you may not— yet. I came to understand holism and what it adds to a healing art very slowly, through years of experiencing different health care choices. So have a number of people. Connie's story at the end of the chapter may illustrate for you the difference a holistic attitude makes, particularly in the midst of a medical crisis.

The holistic point of view sees and experiences a person or thing differently from the Cartesian (or reductionist) perspective. It takes a systemic, complete picture approach. The whole, a system, *is* made up of parts but is something *more than* the sum of its parts. The system is a discrete entity and experience in itself.

For example, a marriage relationship, ideally, is a whole that is more than the sum of its parts, the wife and husband. When both participate to create synergistic blending, there are actually three entities in the marriage. The wife and the husband are each one, with personalities, needs, and experiences of their own. And the relationship has its own qualities that can't be delineated by merely describing the partners together.

The physical, mental, emotional, and spiritual—each dimension represents a different view of the same person. Changes in one catalyze change in other parts of the organism. The mind affects emotions, which affect the body, which affects the spirit, which affects the mind, and so forth.

The new health and medicine movements have adapted holism as an approach to health care. Holistic systems, by design, treat the person as a multidimensional organism in the context of her or his environment. Professionals draw on a variety of health-promoting or curative techniques. These systems are meant to appreciate patients as emotional, mental, social, and spiritual, as well as physical beings.

The Many Meanings of Holistic

People have used, misused, and abused the term *holistic*. People use terms like *alternative medicine, holistic medicine, wellness, and holistic health* interchangeably. It took me time to sort out a general meaning and point of view for these terms for myself. Not everyone is going to agree with my perspective, but this is a multidimensional field in a complex world. I offer you my definitions; that is, until something happens to shift my paradigm!

Alternative Medicine:

Writers, medical doctors, and many healing arts professionals label nonorthodox medicine and health care practices as "alternative." In this case, it means *different* from modern, accepted medicine. People tend to use alternative health practices *instead of* orthodox medicine. Alternative, however, does not guarantee holistic.

Someone may consult an acupuncturist, chiropractor, or naturopathic physician as an alternative to receiving drug therapy or surgery. The degree of holism, or holistic regard for the patient or client, depends on the perspective practiced by the professional—and the patient. Alternative medicines can be used simply to fix a particular condition, as an alternative to the magic pill syndrome. Or they can be used to transform health and lifestyle practices in a more systemic or holistic manner.

Holistic Medicine:

As individual medical doctors awake to possible benefits of some alternative techniques, they begin incorporating them into their medical practices. Holistic medical practices combine orthodox drug and surgery therapies with any number of the more conservative healing arts. Nutrition, meditation or relaxation techniques, exercises or massage, and psychology are popular additions.

The difference is that holistic medicine is just beginning to recognize that there is more than a physical reality and experience to both a disease condition and its treatment. And this perspective still orients activity toward combating illness, rather than achieving health.

Wellness:

Wellness takes the concept of health beyond the mere absence of disease. If a person is sick, wellness practices deal with the disease using a variety of methods. However, the eventual aim is to teach clients to move health from illness to optimum functioning. Clients learn how to change their lifestyle habits from disease-promoting to health-enhancing. The goal: Successful wellness clients are not only disease-free but are also growing, self-actualizing, and feeling good, if not great.

Holistic Health:

Originally a layperson's term used by people not licensed to practice medicine, holistic health is evolving to mean a health *attitude*. Whether an approach is a singular or multidimensional healing art, the professional views the client as a whole organism. Health is treated as an integral aspect of the organism—an entity that is dynamic and constantly changing. Being sick is part of the overall process of living. Illness is not bad. Healing may or may not mean curing a disease and optimum health may or may not be an important goal.

A particular technique or approach may seem to involve only one level of the person; for instance, the physical. However, the practitioner maintains an awareness, respect, and understanding for the interrelatedness of different functional aspects of the client.

Actually, I have found a practitioner's attitude means more than a particular label. I prefer practitioners whose attitudes and regard for clients and client care are truly holistic. A holistic understanding of clients means taking the whole picture of their lives and feelings into consideration, if necessary, when planning a health program.

An Alternative Lion in Holistic Sheepskin

Connie is a diminutive anchor in her friends' lives. She came to JFK University to expand her counseling skills for her astrology practice. Her holistic health studies inspired her to take up volleyball as a form of exercise. One day an aggressive teammate landed on her after spiking a winning point. Connie was knocked out for a few seconds but she carried on for a few days before acknowledging that she had been hurt. She woke up one day in pain, unable to turn her neck.

She called a few friends to find a good chiropractor, and scheduled a session with one. Connie felt assured by the well-appointed, professional environment and holistic health literature in the outer office. The assistant who did the intake interview turned out to be a naturopath practicing under this chiropractor's license. He was patient and compassionate, and he listened to her story. She felt even more assured.

Then the chiropractor made his entrance. Connie describes his Applied Kinesiology muscle-testing evaluation and adjustments as "slam, bam." When he spoke, the chiropractor talked *at* her, not with her. He was entirely uninterested in forming any kind of bond. He didn't inquire about Connie's general well-being nor allay her nervousness. He simply went to work on her. Connie could feel the coldness and indifference in his touch.

The chiropractor told her to sign up for some Hellerwork, one of the adjunct services he offered as part of a comprehensive health care service. Connie paid for the adjustment, walked out of the office, and burst into tears.

While the pain in her neck felt a little bit better, she felt worse.

Needless to say, Connie cancelled the next appointment. She did not want to subject herself further to the insensitive environment and memory of the unholistic chiropractor, no matter how conscious, conscientious, and sensitive all of his staff might have been.

That chiropractor may have been technically brilliant and may have gathered services that seemed holistic under one roof— but he had missed the essential message of holistic care. He did not understand that *how* he does his treatment is as important as, if not more important than, *what* he does.

Complementary Medicine

A holistic attitude includes being able to recognize when a particular healing art may not serve all or enough of a client's health condition or goals. The holistic professional can accept when her client says he wants or needs something else as part of a health care program. This approach to health recognizes the potential relationships between various health care choices, and can include mixing orthodox and nontraditional healing arts.

I regard these practices as "Complementary Medicine"—a term more popular in Great Britain than in America. It expresses the new relationship possible between orthodox medicine and the burgeoning new choices in health lifestyle practices.

The idea of complementary medicine signals a shift from seeing the healing arts as different *and separate* from modern medicine to knowing they can be enhancing and supportive of orthodox treatments. The new health care choices are filling in where medications and surgery may not be appropriate, especially with chronic diseases.

Alternative medicine sounds like "us versus them." Complementary medicine heralds the possibility of "we."

Taking Charge

The holistic health movement is about taking charge of your health care lifestyle. It means self-knowledge and an active sense of accountability for one's own well-being. Knowing yourself, and what it takes for you to be well, helps you live your daily life in a health-enhancing way.

Tom Ferguson was an eager Yale Medical School student, getting his first taste of clinical medicine. He was surprised and disappointed at how many partially or totally *preventable* diseases he saw on his rounds. For instance, he saw smokers with lung cancer and heart disease, and sedentary fat men struck down by heart attacks. People came in with physical symptoms that were really about job, relationship, or money problems.

Whether these patients suffered from lack of information or motivation, Ferguson wanted to do something to change the situation. In the late '70s, he started a magazine and assembled a book, *Medical Self-Care,* to educate people to prevent and treat common problems themselves. Ferguson and others, such as his friend John Travis, M.D. (Wellness Resource Center), are part of a growing number of health professionals working to make laypeople more aware and self-sufficient as health clients.

Participating Health Clients versus Passive Patients

Health clients participate in their own self-care by establishing ongoing partnerships with one or more health care profession-

9

als to create good health. Unlike some refugees from insensitive medical care, conscious health clients do not stubbornly or defensively try to go it alone. They choose a primary care provider as a guide, or as a home base while they try various other healing arts.

They build a professional "team" and seek support from family, friends, and community for facing health challenges. Participating clients are less likely to go overboard searching for self-care techniques or alternative medicine.

Finally, they understand that consulting a professional creates a relationship. Participating clients take an active role in the five stages of working with a health professional.

These clients choose to avoid high-risk behaviors. For instance, they minimize major contributors to illness or chronic conditions, such as excessive drinking, smoking, overwork, poor nutrition, and overeating. They also participate in health-enhancing activities, such as good nutrition, exercise, rest, and relaxation.

Equally important, they take care to avoid passive health-related behavior. A typical passive patient neglects his health until he gets sick. He may complain about the stress in his everyday life, but he ignores what it is doing to him psychologically, emotionally, and physically. He raises his blood pressure and cholesterol with rich, heavy meals or he risks cancer by smoking. Perhaps he strains his nerves and immune system with late nights at the office.

Finally, his body cries "enough!" He collapses and arrives at the doctor's office or the hospital, feeling helpless, angry, victimized. Some passive patients are even mystified at how this could happen to them.

A passive patient surrenders the responsibility for getting well to others. His attitude is "Fix me up, Doc." Raised on the idea that there is a magic pill for just about anything, the passive patient wants the doctor to stop the pain, to just make this crisis go away.

The participating health client consciously works to reduce the odds for arriving at the hospital needing to "be fixed." He has changed his lifestyle to prevent many of the typical stress-related medical crises.

Becoming a participating health client starts with evaluating your needs, goals, or problems. Then you decide how much and what kind of help you require in changing your health lifestyle. The next step is establishing a relationship with the person or persons who are going to be your resources, guides, and service providers.

The Primary Care Provider

A participating health client often finds a primary health care provider. In the U.S. most states legally define primary health care professionals as those who provide first line treatment consultations and access to health insurance billing. It varies by state, but the list can include medical doctors, naturopathic physicians, chiropractors, dentists, osteopaths, and certified acupuncturists.

A primary care provider acts as monitor and interpreter, as well as a health service provider. He recognizes pain and other signs or symptoms as signals, and the human body as a system. He knows your medical history, the overview of your health situation, and the various treatments or activities in which you are engaged. As a monitor, he can prevent different treatments or healing arts from negating each other's effects—or reacting to each other with harmful or toxic effects.

News stories began appearing in the late '80s about over-medicated senior citizens. Many older people see more than one doctor for the multiple problems that accompany old age and deteriorating health. They often get one or more prescriptions from each physician. Some patients interviewed had been taking 15 to 21 different pills every day with ineffective or deadly results. No one, least of all the patient, was keeping track. Medical authorities now call on seniors to have a primary care physician, one who will be informed about the various specialists consulted and the different medications prescribed.

Everyone under multiple treatment needs someone to keep an overview—and to confirm the necessity and efficacy of any component interacting in the total picture. The primary care professional knows his patient's "baseline health" before any crisis. He keeps the client appraised of her ongoing health conditions and needs. He is someone with whom to share ideas about adding complementary healing arts to a health care program. He can provide perspective, direction, information, warning, and possible alternatives for a self-generated health program.

For the independent health seeker, interested in trying the latest in healing arts, the primary care provider can be an anchor, advising on contraindications to any suggested complementary services. Most of all, he can check that the eager or ambitious client does not do too much at once. Too much of anything can yield unproductive results.

Going Overboard

Self-exploration and self-awareness can be heady experiences. Bodywork provides contact for the touch starved; counseling, a captive audience for those who feel ignored. Taking charge of one's health can feel really good.

On the other hand, small victories over chronic problems may precipitate perplexing relapses or new problems. As physical health changes, whether for better or worse, it can stir up unfamiliar emotions and long buried memories. Taking charge can be confusing.

I have talked with many people during my pursuits of self-help, holistic health, bodywork, psychotherapy, metaphysics, and "new age" marketing. Along the way, I noticed some individuals going overboard in their search. The American culture seems to promote the idea that if a little is good, more is better. People may be driven, desperately seeking answers for their misery. Or, they may drift from one good idea or attractive activity to another, experimenting with new healing techniques and spiritual philosophies without real goals or direction.

Sometimes I hear a person described as having "gone off the deep end" with "all that holistic stuff" or "that Shirley Mac-Laine craziness." To the uninitiated, it seems that fervent seekers often lose themselves in the search. And, indeed, some seekers *may* lose sight of themselves or their original goals.

For instance, "bodywork junkies" sign up for class after class, go from massage technician to body therapist looking for contact and release. They are hoping that pushing the right muscles back in place, crying enough tears from dredged-up memories, or feeling the caring touch of a compassionate healer will solve life's problems. While all these experiences may help, they may avoid addressing the real underlying causes for their distress—stress from family relationships, work, nutrition, or their own psychological and emotional makeup.

Then there are the "health detectives," caught up in the game of figuring out what's really wrong with themselves. Each new technique gives them another piece of the puzzle. Making connections between health conditions and lifestyles, traumatic incidents and muscle knots, or psychological issues and behavioral problems is stimulating. The investigation becomes the purpose, and the goal is ignored. To solve the puzzle stops the play, so the search—and the health problem—goes on.

Finally, I notice "spiritual escapees." They are today's affluent flower children, who spread their unconditional love with symbols, such as crystals, astrology, tarot, and runes. They often try to manage their health using the powers of the mind or the spirit realm. Escapees might try tying a crystal over a throat that is beginning to feel sore. Sometimes it works, but not always.

In the normal, cyclical nature of health, getting "sick" may be natural, even necessary, for the body to regain equilibrium. Or pain or fever can signal something more serious, something that needs professional attention.

Whatever their potential uses, tools and talismans need to be kept in proper perspective. The caution is to make sure you are not using the metaphysical or the symbolic to avoid facing what is really going on with feelings or the physical body.

Staying on the Right Track

Searching for health solutions in a compulsive or scattered way can put the original problem or goal out of focus. It disorganizes a health plan, and dissipates direction. By setting off in the wrong direction, do-it-yourself health seekers can mask serious problems with partial solutions, and delay inevitable health crises that would force them to get the help they need. Here is where a primary care provider can be of enormous value.

Frank Shallenberger, M.D. sees a number of refugees from self-care routines. Some, like me, may have food sensitivities that are out of control. They originally dropped out of orthodox medical care because of insensitive physicians or narrow treatment perspectives. They have tried anything from acupuncture and energy balancing to muscle testing and elimination diets. Often they have come to limit their diet to two or three foodstuffs. They are desperate.

Shallenberger looks at a wide variety of issues from several different perspectives. He checks for thyroid function, a compromised immune system, metabolic deficiencies, and the possibility of candida or other chronic conditions. He listens to each patient's story, paying particular attention to contributing stress factors.

Shallenberger recommends several different treatment modalities. Like most primary care providers, his overview and access to diagnostics and treatment resources completely outstrips what do-it-yourself health nuts can do for themselves. For holistic health–oriented clients, he is willing to listen to and comment on their ideas about adding complementary healing arts to a health plan or treatment program. More and more doctors today are beginning to adopt Shallenberger's approach, and the concept of consulting with clients to give them an overview of available resources (case management) has arrived on the orthodox health scene.

David Zimmerman, a licensed counselor and teacher in Santa Cruz, is creating one kind of case management niche. He focuses on holistic health seekers whose health problems cause emotional stress. Zimmerman helps them choose healing arts that may aid their search for physical balance and release, enhance functioning despite a crippling chronic condition, or return to normal— whatever their goal.

Typically, even when health seekers focus only on their physical challenges, psychological problems arise as well. Bodywork, for one, stirs up repressed emotions and potentially painful memories. Using his "Catalytic Intervention" concepts, Zimmerman guides clients through intense psychoemotional therapy and advises them on various healing arts that they may choose to complement their mental and physical healing processes. He teaches them how to articulate their needs and specific requests to a bodyworker. And he helps them process and integrate information and emotions that come out of the body therapy sessions.

Zimmerman also works with health practitioners to help them define their scope of practice. He teaches them to recognize clients in distress, those who need more counseling than just the friendly and compassionate attention of a massage technician. Often a client who has pulled away from orthodox health services may mistakenly expect a certain kind of care from health workers not trained to handle that specific need. The practitioner learns to keep informed about alternative or complementary health care choices, and to accept when a client requires something outside her field and recommend seeking other help.

Change can be difficult. It can be scary. Self-responsibility takes courage, because taking charge of your health, your life, and your lifestyle means learning new behaviors. We learned to be the way we are; we learned the lifestyle habits and beliefs that may stress our health. We can unlearn them, too.

The rewards for taking charge of our health, and for seeking out and accepting appropriate support for this process, are more than just better health. Participating health clients discover new feelings about themselves and new ways of seeing and experiencing health.

A New Generation of Practitioners

◇ **T**he holistic health practitioners you meet today walk a narrow path between the dominant orthodox medicine and the alternative lifestyle fringes. They are breaking ground, defining a place for themselves as professionals in the health care field and bringing wider choices to society. At the same time, medical doctors are becoming more open to a holistic philosophy. Together, sometimes at the insistence of their clients and patients, these health care workers are making a new generation of professionals.

Like their clients, most holistic practitioners are seekers. Being a marriage of Western and Eastern medicines, the holistic health movement has opened new cultural and philosophical horizons. The new practitioners acknowledge that healing involves more than any one particular technique. Practitioners' tools, language, and approaches to their health care services often reflect this new consciousness. More intimacy, more real caring is possible, adding to the healing process.

Bodyworkers and counselors are helping clients heal deep physical, emotional, and spiritual wounds. Many professional health care providers integrate Chinese or Indian medicine-based philosophy or Buddhist spiritual principles into a Western health approach. Doctors who are otherwise conservative draw on the power of the mind as part of a treatment plan in Behavioral Medicine.

The Pioneers

The new holistic professionals are the intellectual, spiritual, and technical descendants of healing arts pathfinders and pioneers throughout history. With single-minded purposefulness, the pioneers pursued their visions or reintroduced ancient knowledge to the health marketplace.

The second section of this book, which profiles various healing arts, includes many examples of the new health pioneers. Their work spans more than 100 years. Some have combined modern knowledge and their own original insights into completely new technologies. Others have helped to establish age-old medical and healing wisdom, such as Ayurveda and shamanism, in our modern society.

For example, Alyce and Elmer Green helped establish Biofeedback as both a healing and research tool. They continue to test the latest healing modalities, such as the channeling of "bioenergy." Edward Bach's experiments expanded homeopathic medicines into the spiritual-emotional realm of Flower Essences and Remedies. And David Palmer ignored critics as he developed Chiropractic in the late 1800s and early 1900s.

Graduates of the human potential movement, mavericks in orthodox medicine, and laypersons with insights on how the human being works—all may be inventing new healing modalities at this moment. Holistic health is a growing, dynamic field.

Most pioneers and pathfinders develop their points of view with almost fanatical effort. For instance, F. M. Alexander watched himself in a three-way mirror to understand his posture and balance and their effects on his voice. He worked with himself this way for nine years to create the Alexander Technique.

Once a new system, approach, or point of view is firmly established, the pioneer often launches a public tour. Grateful clients spread word of the benefits of the new approach. Public interest and professional acceptance of the work is tested on the lecture circuit, earning successful pioneers popularity and notoriety.

Sooner or later the Randolph Stones and Ida Rolfs write books about Polarity or Rolfing, recording their findings and establishing their systems' integrity. Appointments with the now well-known master are prized. Going to the source of a popular healing modality may mean being kept on a long waiting list or paying a premium price.

Apprentices then carry on the pioneer's work. As the leader ages or the healing art's popularity expands, students organize an institute or association to take over its teaching, promotion, and preservation. Top graduates train the next generation of practitioners, freeing the originator to write, lecture, and concentrate on advanced students.

Philosophical differences can develop. Judith Aston and Joseph Heller separately moved out of the shadow of Ida Rolf to create their own therapeutic bodyworks. Both added new perspectives and original techniques to the Structural Integration pioneered by Rolf. Aston and Heller, in turn, are training their next generations of practitioners.

The Settlers

You and I, as health consumers, are more likely to see second- and third-generation holistic professionals. They are the current creators of the holistic health movement. Like the settlers of the Old West who established communities in territories opened by pioneering pathfinders, this new generation of practitioners is carving out a new health territory and marketplace, and establishing a relationship between formerly "alternative" health care techniques and mainstream America.

It's a tricky business. Often practitioners or their professional organizations must lobby and negotiate through choppy political and legal waters, fend off public skepticism or media exploitation, and continue to educate potential clients about the benefits of their particular healing arts.

Yet a majority of the next generation's professionals are working almost anonymously to prove the value of their new techniques to a critical mass of clients and supporters. And in the everyday practice of their science and art, some healers are finding new ways to use their knowledge. They begin to pioneer new techniques and approaches to help clients meet health challenges. And the creative process continues, catalyzed and crystallized by the relationship between practitioner and client.

The patient/client and the doctor/practitioner need to be engaged together in the healing process in order to create a partnership. Participation and partnership reap rewards for both the patient and the practitioner. Both learn, change, grow. The practitioner helps the client achieve her health goal. The client, in turn, gives the practitioner a new healing experience. In this way, the client becomes part of the entire holistic odyssey, helping other health care seekers down the road by helping the practitioner hone his healing art.

A Healing Beyond Surgery

Laura, a friend of mine, was referred to a top surgeon for a complex and perplexing gynecological condition. The surgeon was the medical detective she needed, and the swift intervention of orthodox medicine was probably the best or only solution. However, Laura was concerned because she assumed he was a "straight" doctor rather than "holistic." Although she was in crisis and scared, she stubbornly toyed with seeking alternative treatment. Still, she kept her appointment with the physician—just in case.

It was a transformational experience. She did her best to manage her fear and panic, listened to the doctor's evaluation, and asked for time to think over the options and prepare for possible surgery. The doctor told her how much time she could responsibly take. She spent two weeks discussing the options and her feelings with her therapist. She meditated and talked with friends to decide what she could do, should it come to surgery, to deal with the feelings of helplessness and victimization.

All along, Laura and the doctor kept talking and taking further tests. Since surgeons are used to being in charge and my friend can be quite independent and stubborn, a few of those consultations were undoubtedly a bit like tug-of-war. However, when time was up and the doctor told her she had to make her decision, she went to the hospital with a sense of relief. She had developed a deep trust for the surgeon and for her ability to cope with the consequences of a worst-case scenario. She and the doctor had established a bond of communication, mutual respect, and partnership in the healing process.

The surgeon was very flexible. Or perhaps he was responding to her intention to participate in the healing process. Laura decided she needed to wear a Walkman to play music before, during, and after the operation, to have a crystal taped in the palm of one hand, and to bring her stuffed bear to watch over her in the operating room.

The doctor cleared it with the hospital and probably took some ribbing from the other doctors about his weird patient. But that was how Laura wanted to face this operation. He could see that and was willing to break hospital rules and smudge his professional image for her sake. That is a healing partnership.

The story—and benefits—of this doctor/patient healing partnership continue. Two years later, Laura was still bothered that she had been given an amnesia-inducing drug before surgery. She was upset at losing her memory and not knowing where she had been in the hospital. The surgeon arranged for her to suit up in the hospital greens and took her step by step through the prep, operating, and recovery rooms to ease and satisfy her mind. What a gift—and recognition of the patient as a whole person.

A healing partnership emphasizes self-responsibility and self-exploration. Both the professional and the client endeavor to learn and grow from their interaction. That bond of mutual support, respect, and learning begins from the very first interaction, the first interview or appointment.

What Makes a Good Practitioner

Masseuse or dentist, acupuncturist or M.D., the professional brings very human qualities to the client-practitioner relationship. In a healing partnership—a helping relationship—the helper is more alike than different from the "helpee."

The patient and the professional have all their human attributes in common. Psychotherapist Lawrence Brammer, in *The Helping Relationship,* talks about the qualities a client and a therapist bring to the first interview appointment, which is similar to a first consultation with any health care professional. His list illustrates the point that there is only one main difference between the "helpee" and the helper.

Helpee	Helper
self-perceptions	self-perceptions
values	values
feelings	feelings
experiences	experiences
expectations	expectations
problems	*expertise*

It is that one main difference, the patient's problem and professional's expertise, that brings them together. They make contact and forge a relationship for the purpose of an exchange.

This human bond makes the relationship. Relationships are dynamic, changing, living processes, created by what each participant brings to them. The relationship becomes greater than the sum of its parts, adding to the healing process.

A mark of a good practitioner is a conscious realization that she is part of a system, a partner in the healing process. She brings parts of herself to the helping process, is open and available. And at the same time she takes care of herself, participates in the relationship with appropriate boundaries.

Boundaries, in counseling and holistic circles, means knowing where you end and the rest of the world begins. It means being sensitive to times when you might be breaching another person's personal and emotional space.

Good health care professionals give of themselves without giving up more time, energy, or intimacy than they can comfortably handle. They know the difference between touching and penetrating, between relating and overwhelming, between meeting someone on her own ground and draining her with overattentiveness.

The aware or conscious practitioner can also sense when it is appropriate not to be therapeutic, but just to perform the technique instead. Many new health care customers are not used to the intimacy and contact of a therapeutic relationship. Some come to a masseur just for a massage. That's okay. Whether this is an optimal treatment or not, it is all that is desired. A good practitioner can respect those limits. It is part of respecting each client.

A sense of partnership in the healing relationship is only one element that elevates a professional beyond being a capable technician. We expect high quality education and proven competence in the professionals we consult.

Continually updating skills and knowledge is another mark of a conscientious therapist, doctor, or practitioner. Innate talent, an intuitive awareness or feel for the client and the work, and wisdom gained from experience—all add special qualities to the consultation or session.

However, having people skills—empathy, friendliness, warmth—and emphasizing participation by both the client and professional are what make the difference between a competent practitioner and one who stands out as "good." And as a client, your ability to participate with that practitioner can make the difference in how—and how well—the professional can help you.

Bringing Out the Best in Each Other

In a healing partnership, a professional's qualities and abilities are enhanced when matched by the client's ability to ask for and respond to them. It is important to speak up and say what you need and want, what you think and feel. Your ability to ask questions and listen supports the professional's willingness and ability to communicate his findings and recommendations, to give you the fullest explanation you require.

At the same time, you can maximize your primary care provider's ability to listen and gather data by organizing your thoughts and saying succinctly what is on your mind at any consultation. One study by a Wayne State University doctor showed that medical doctors interrupt their patients' answers to their first question after about 18 seconds and spend only an average of three minutes with each person.

Being open and nonjudgmental makes a comfortable atmosphere in which both you and the professional can exchange information. Clients sometimes have fears and intimate details to share that are important to the treatment process or their own healing experience. The professional's ability to accept you allows you to reveal that which may be hard to talk about to others.

The same is true for your regard for the professional. Practitioners cannot be all things to all people. Your expectations must be realistic. Your acceptance of their humanity gives them the room to feel, learn, explore, rather than try to live up to the role of God.

My friend, Laura, told me the ultimate reward of her surgery was something her surgeon said after it was all over. He remarked at their final follow-up appointment that she was the easiest patient he had ever worked with, because she took responsibility for herself. He recognized her partnership in the treatment program and this made it fun for him. He did not feel the load was all dumped on him, nor did he feel the threat of blame if things did not turn out as expected.

Laura's acceptance of the surgeon as a human being with top-notch expertise gave him the room to explore his own limits of how he wants to practice medicine. Over the years, they have continued to exchange healing information. He helped her confront certain problems caused by her being an adult child of alcoholics and encouraged her to seek help for overeating—even though neither area was strictly in the realm of his medical practice.

Accepting a practitioner as a person and respecting his expertise includes allowing him to not know everything. It takes maturity, security, and self-confidence for an expert to say "I don't know" to a question or situation. Not knowing offers the opportunity to find out—the chance for a dialogue between you and your expert. That exploration and dialogue can be a creative partnership and part of the healing process.

Participating in a Health Care Relationship— The Five Stages

Whether using orthodox medicine, so-called alternative medicine, or complementary health practices, there are five stages of a healing partnership:

Choosing a Professional: selecting the type of health care and a particular practitioner.

Information Exchange: giving history and goals, receiving feedback, asking and answering questions.

Planning and Deciding: listening to options and recommendations from the professional, working on making the decision, deciding together what to do.

Doing It, Follow-up, and Support: the actual work of the health care program, maintaining communication during the process, gathering emotional and other kinds of support.

Endings and Closure: tying up loose ends of information and feelings to understand your final status, hearing and saying what you need to complete the experience.

There are particular responsibilities that you can adopt to maximize your health care at each stage of the relationship. The role you take in any healing program depends on your goals. Losing 20 pounds demands very different levels of participation on your part than dealing with a broken leg. The role you take also depends on the type of healing art you choose. Medical history-taking and session planning for a series of Rolfings, for example, is much different than for a series of Traditional Chinese Medicine treatments.

The role your health care practitioner takes also depends on the circumstances. Nevertheless, during each stage of the relationship, there are special attributes and qualities desirable in a helping professional.

Stage One: Choosing a Professional

Faced with a task beyond our understanding or expertise, we learn to call in help. We take our car to an auto mechanic, our taxes to an accountant. Choosing expert help is an important beginning. It sets the tone for everything that follows.

The most important factor in choosing health professionals is the match between their skills and your problem or goals. Being clear about what you need and want helps narrow the choices. It gives you clear-cut questions to ask the practitioner during the initial phase of the search.

There are several other attributes to seek in a health care professional before you make an introductory appointment:

☐ She should be willing to be interviewed, at least by phone.

☐ She should answer (or have the staff answer) questions about:
- training and certification
- the scope of practice, specialties, and special interests
- her methods of assessment and treatment
- the use of tests, medications, supplements, and other material (she should understand if you have lots of allergies)
- the kind of information required for medical history

☐ She should have a staff that is supportive, articulate, and enthusiastic.

☐ Her fees, location, and availability should fit your lifestyle.

Stage Two: Information Exchange

You know the routine. You sit in the outer office, waiting to see the doctor, filling out forms with family medical history along with the all-important insurance information. Some acupuncture and homeopathic clinics use similar questionnaires as shortcuts to getting basic data.

However, as the client, your role is not only to provide answers to the professional's questions but also to state your goals and to ask about what you don't understand. How or how well a practitioner answers is another thing. There are several qualities that a healing professional should display during this stage:

❏ She should ask open-ended questions, giving you a chance to say what is on your mind, why you are there, and what you want.

❏ She should listen to you.

❏ She should keep you focused on the purpose of the visit but not limit the scope of the conversation unduly.

❏ She should make you feel comfortable.

❏ She should draw out the information she needs for assessment with patience and, hopefully, a little humor.

❏ She should meet any fear or resistance on your part with a minimum of defensiveness on her part.

❏ She should offer perspective, information, expertise, and options—not pronouncements, "truths," or orders.

❏ She should answer all your questions, even if the answer is "I don't know."

❏ She should be willing to share the discovery process.

❏ She should be willing to explain why she wants to know something and how it relates to your case.

❏ She should be honest, her actions matching her words and attitude.

Stage Three: Planning and Deciding

Listening and analytical skills come in handy at this stage. Your role here is to ask questions and give feedback about whatever the provider proposes for treatment or course of action. Then you must decide for yourself. In a complex health challenge, if you are fortunate you will be able to choose from among several options. Simple healing arts can also provide options and choice. In a complex health situation, your practitioner's role is multifaceted:

❑ She should offer options, and explain the pros and cons of each one.

❑ She should give details about her recommendations—how they are to be carried out and by whom.

❑ She should give the cost of each option, if applicable.

❑ She should answer all questions until you understand.

❑ She should give you a chance to discuss ideas, voice fears, and make your own suggestions.

❑ She should be sensitive to your need for time to think and decide—and communicate how much time is appropriate according to the situation (emergencies have very different pressures and timeliness for treatment than chronic conditions).

❑ She should explain possible consequences or side effects of the healing art or treatment modality.

❑ She should be aware of and articulate her biases about options, feelings, or issues in any approach.

❑ She should be open to your desire to seek another opinion, other options, or additional support.

You have the right to ask the practitioner anything regarding what is recommended or asked of you. It helps you participate in planning and deciding on activites in a complex or long-term health care program. It engages you and contributes to your motivation to follow the recommended course of treatment, to make a series of lifestyle changes, or just to be present at each consultation or therapy session.

Stage Four: Doing It, Follow-up, And Support

This is it. Now you have to do it. Showing up for a massage is one thing, changing eating and exercise habits is another. Taking an active role in a healing program involves putting your time, energy, and self on the line.

It goes better with support. Don't be afraid to check in with your practitioner on the progress you have made, or call to clarify some instructions.

You should expect your health care provider to follow up during a long-term health-enhancing plan:

❏ She should make herself available for questions or discussion.

❏ She should set up a schedule for follow-up evaluation.

❏ She should be clear about when she is available (for example, "My answering service will put a call through after office hours in a crisis").

❏ She should continue to keep you appraised of her evaluation of your progress.

❏ She should alert you to changes that have occurred in you, the treatment program, or your case, and explain their meaning.

❏ She should remain open to your adding other healing arts and practitioners and be willing to listen to and share information on these other support activities.

❏ She should be able to recommend support groups, when applicable, or other sources of information.

Your primary care provider, however, is not your only resource. Building a support network, especially when you have to make big changes in your life, is important. It is good to have one or more people available for "reality checks." They should be family or friends who know you, your life situation, and your health. Their role is to tell you what they observe—their perceptions and understanding of what you are doing and how they see it affecting you.

Stage Five: Endings and Closure

There are two basic endings to a healing partnership. One is the natural conclusion of a plan or task, when a goal is accomplished. The other is an interruption in treatment because one or both parties are dissatisfied with the situation or service. Tying up details and saying good-bye is much easier in the first case. Telling someone that she is not fulfilling expectations is hard.

It is up to both the health client and practitioner to bring a situation and relationship to a satisfying end. This means anything from walking away with just a thank-you and good-bye to a detailed conversation about the treatment and outcome. Some clients request copies of their records. I usually ask to exchange a hug as a good-bye.

As a healing program ends—or you decide to terminate the relationship—the health care professional has certain responsibilities:

❏ She should give you a final evaluation of your case.

❏ She should be willing to give you copies of your records, including test results, notes, and the final evaluation.

❏ She should be willing to listen to your reasons for ending the relationship if other than the natural conclusion of treatment or a health process. (This can be difficult when your needs have not been met.)

❏ She should say to you what she needs or wants to say (and you must be willing to listen—even if she tells you that you are making a mistake and why).

❏ She should leave the door open for you to return if you need and want to.

If the experience was upsetting or unsatisfactory in any way, it is up to you whether you need to communicate that to the professional, the staff, or any authority. Personal style or personality clash is one thing. Incompetence is another.

Connie, the woman who had the bad chiropractic experience, braved talking to that abrupt chiropractor over the phone after she cancelled follow-up appointments with his office. Despite pleasant interactions with his support staff, she told him, his manner offended her and got in the way of any healing effects of his technique. He allowed that they had different personal styles but never really apologized.

Connie still tells this story, some five years later, with a certain amount of emotion. However, taking a stand, asserting herself to get out of an unpleasant health care service, and confronting the offending practitioner were big steps in her personal development. She strengthened her stance as a health client and changed how she took care of herself.

Ready for the Adventure to Begin?

I have talked about this new idea, the holistic health movement. I pointed out some of the different ways of thinking about health and some of the pitfalls of diving into a new "paradigm." I stressed the importance of having a primary care provider as a guide or home base as you venture out into new health territory. And I discussed the opportunity for creating a healing partnership with your practitioners throughout the health care relationship.

The next step is exploring for yourself the new options for creating your health care lifestyle. The following chapter, *The Healing Spiral,* is a discovery map—a way to look at all the different, new healing arts available.

The Healing Spiral

 ## The Spiral Metaphor

The image of the spiral appears over and over again in nature, art, and mythology. Open a nautilus shell and see its outwardly spiraling chambers, reminding us of the expansive patterns in life. Read in the Bible about the builders of the Tower of Babel who tried to wind their way to heaven. Watch water go down a drain.

The spiral is a universal form that symbolizes dynamic motion around a fixed point. Spirals can descend in decreasing space, ascend in ever-expanding reach, or proceed along a continuum in an even, cylindrical way.

So can the healing journey.

Orthodox medicine retains the mythical caduceus as its symbol. Two snakes, representing human energy rising toward enlightenment, spiral around a wing-topped staff. This was the staff used by the Greek god Hermes to guide souls to rebirth. The journey toward both enlightenment and health is circular, around a central, anchoring, and guiding path. I see the healing journey as a spiral revolving around an essential core of who we are.

The spiral is a way to imagine an experience of the whole self. It is hard to be aware of all of our self, all at once. Try thinking of how the bottom of your feet feel against your shoes, listening to the sound and rhythm of your breathing, and looking at a thumbnail—all at once. Now, at the same time try remembering yesterday's shopping, visualizing a tender moment you want to have with a loved one, and eating dinner. Difficult, no?

31

The spiral also describes a movement through changes in life and health. For me it symbolizes a rhythm, a pulse of life as I progress through chronological time and the evolution of my health. I move between focusing on different issues, different parts of my health, different phases of wellness.

All the while, each new realization and experience adds up to more total awareness. Like the proverbial peeling of an onion, I discover more and more layers of my experience. I gain understanding of myself as a complex, multileveled human system. As I progress toward a more holistic experience, I translate that awareness to my approach to health. For instance, I've finally realized and accepted that my body is not the enemy. I no longer think and speak of my physical body as "it" but rather as "me."

And as I flow from a level of relative health to a level of seeming illness, I visualize it as progress. Each period of feeling "not well" is less alarming and more informative. The "healing crisis" or sickness is a message, a signal that my body is taking a natural course of action to rid itself of pollutants or imbalances.

I know how to use each challenge as an opportunity to grow and change. Each period of "feeling good" is at a higher or more solid plateau. My health focus has expanded past the crises of rampant food allergies to vaster realms of my life—my work, values, friends and community, faith in life, and purpose for being alive. This is my holistic experience.

Holism, remember, describes an individual's health as a dynamic interaction between all aspects of human beingness. Physical health is only one component. Holistic health also takes into account the psychoemotional, community, familial, and spiritual influences and consequences. Accessing one level affects all the others to one degree or another.

One can only go so far in developing health by concentrating on only one or two aspects. At some point, progress slows, stops, or even relapses if other aspects of human health are neglected or rejected.

The man recovering from a heart attack can change his diet, take medication religiously, and follow a sensible exercise routine. He may even force himself to slow down at work. However, if he does not transform his "Type A" emotions—anger and a sense that there isn't enough time—these pressured attitudes will infuse every action. His values and choices remain stuck in the old pattern. He may begin to exercise to excess or to alienate family support with his emotional outbursts. Medication and diet can only do so much to keep his blood pressure down. And as he feels the new pattern of health eroding, he is likely to allow old patterns of defense to creep back into his behavior. The new man begins to fade back into the picture of the old.

The journey to wellness is not a straight line. Along the way, there may be some stalls, jumps ahead, or even some U-turns. However, the sum total of all levels of experience adds up to a spiraling one way or the other. The choice of which direction to take is yours. You make that choice by choosing to change.

Tools for Change: Complementary Healing Arts Characteristics and Goals

The tools to make a change in your health are out there. More are being created every day. The holistic health field is a spiral itself. You stand on the outside looking in, knowing you want to start somewhere. It may be a bit overwhelming. There is no opening, no obvious entry point or right place to start.

My purpose is to give you as a healing arts explorer a handle on the door to the new health field. Remember, one healing art is not necessarily going to do it all for you.

The following lists represent different views on the basic healing arts covered in the book. First, I divided them into two divisions by scope of practice. The four Primary Care systems take an overview approach. The rest of the healing arts take more specific aim on health conditions.

Some are named under several headings because many healing arts have a range of benefits, goals, and styles. Start with the benefits you seek and then read the chapters to decide where to take your first slice out of the holistic health field.

Scope of Practice

Scope of practice means how much of a human being and variety of health problems the practice or the practitioner can address. Within many medical systems, different practitioners may have different scopes of practice. In modern Western medicine, the scope ranges from a wide general practice, such as family medicine, down to a narrow specialization, like neurosurgery or gynecology.

Primary Care

HEALTH OVERVIEWS

❑ Acupuncture and Traditional Chinese Medicine

❑ Ayurveda

❑ Chiropractic, Osteopathy and Other Manipulative Arts

❑ Homeopathy

❑ Naturopathic Medicine

Certain cultures and individuals have created a systemic approach to health care from detailed empirical studies of both the body and the tools of each particular system. The actual scope of an individual's practice may be limited, not involving the total resources and view of the system. However, primary care health services are bodies of knowledge that have an over-view.

While they vary by state in America and by country in the rest of the world, medical systems or systemic approaches to health care are classified as "primary care" medicine. This means they are a place to begin in dealing with a health care challenge or goal. In countries with health insurance systems, they are also the entry point into the reimbursement maze.

For example, the point of entry into our Western medical system is the generalist who then may refer certain problems to a specialist. Some states recognize other primary care services, such as chiropractic, naturopathic medicine, and acupuncture. And in many places, M.D.s combine their acute care medical skills with Ayurvedic counseling, acupuncture, or homeopathic practices.

Choosing a primary care healing art is a shotgun approach, covering a wide target of resources, needs or goals. Different overview or systemic healing arts handle the various health aspects of human beings in different ways.

In Western culture, doctors are trained to focus primarily on our anatomical and biochemical levels or systems. Psychiatry, Western medicine's approach to human psychoemotional problems, is a separate specialization. On the other hand, the philosophical foundations of Ayurvedic medicine include both spiritual and psychological concerns. Ayurvedic assessment of physical symptoms incorporates an individual's temperament and environmental relationship. Yet another system, the English or Worsley school of Traditional Chinese Medicine, includes emotional correlations to acupuncture energy meridians.

Along with modern or allopathic medicine, the West developed four more primary care systems: Chiropractic, Homeopathy, Naturopathic Medicine, and Osteopathy. Homeopathic and naturopathic practices are more accepted in Europe, where they were first developed. Chiropractic and osteopathy, founded by Americans, have taken root here.

The systemic healing arts can be used for both acute care or long-term health building goals. The strength of each one varies in addressing conditions that range from emergency to chronic. Homeopathy is on the rise in America due to its successes in dealing with chronic or long-term conditions that orthodox, allopathic medicine fails to cure. Chiropractic care often gets back pain patients to work faster and more cost-effectively than orthodox medical treatment.

Modern Western medicine's technological approach to emergency care is recognized as superior. However, while strong on crisis management, allopathy is weak on patient education. One must search for the right practitioners or health insurance systems in Western medicine to find support for general health maintenance concerns. Wellness education and preventative medical practices, such as well-baby centers, are a specialized branch of orthodox allopathic medicine, not the norm.

Beyond Primary Care

Most health clients start with a problem and then look for the right healing art to solve it. Orthodox or other primary care medicines may not be the most appropriate or effective tools for a particular condition. There are complementary healing arts that take more specific aim at the human health process.

It is a client's market, with many different approaches and styles from which to choose. Various healing arts demand different levels of training and competence. Some have home remedy or self-care routines or products. Often, entry-level classes are available for laypeople.

The majority of these healing arts address the physical body. However, some also integrate the mind, try to effect change in mental-emotional aspects, or include in their approach and outlook a recognition of the spiritual dimension.

TOUCH AND RELAXATION
- ❏ Massage
- ❏ Reflexology
- ❏ Rosen Method
- ❏ Trager
- ❏ Acupressure

The first group of physical healing arts uses direct touch of the body, a gentle manipulation of muscles or soft tissue. These techniques offer experiences that range from relaxing and nurturing to energizing. Some are done on clients who are undressed (draped in towels or sheets); many practitioners use oils or lotions. While the pressure or stroke may contact tight or sore muscle knots, it should not intrude into the body enough to cause any pain.

MANIPULATION AND RESTRUCTURING
- ❏ Alexander Technique
- ❏ Chiropractic, Osteopathy, and other Manipulative Arts
- ❏ Myotherapy
- ❏ Rolfing

The goal of these arts is to correct structural, postural, and/or balance problems. They work on the relationship between body parts, focusing on muscles, joints, or bone alignment. These techniques are interventive. They can intrude into the body and sometimes cause temporary pain. While there is responsiveness to individual differences, the manipulative arts have an idea of what is normal and work to make you fit that picture.

ENERGETIC BALANCE
- ❏ Acupressure
- ❏ Acupuncture and Traditional Chinese Medicine
- ❏ Bach and Flower Essences
- ❏ Healers
- ❏ Homeopathy
- ❏ Polarity
- ❏ Reiki
- ❏ Reflexology
- ❏ Therapeutic Touch

These perspectives recognize the subtle energy interactions between aspects of the client, and between the client, environment, and practitioner. They are based on Eastern energy meridian maps or Western ideas of bioenergy or energetic zones. Practitioners usually talk about *chi, prana,* or electromagnetic energy. Clients are normally clothed during sessions, including those healing arts which are bodyworks.

In his book, *Vibrational Medicine*, Richard Gerber, M.D. calls this health field Einsteinian medicine. He contrasts the relativistic approach of these perspectives with the dominant Western medicine cause-and-effect approach to disease. Its focus is to affect the underlying factors in symptoms or imbalances by moving, unblocking, or balancing energy throughout the physical, energetic, or spirit bodies.

MOVEMENT AND EXERCISE
❑ T'ai Chi, Aikido, and other Martial Arts
❑ Rolf Movement
❑ Rosen Movement
❑ Trager Mentastic
❑ Yoga

For health explorers looking to integrate regular exercise or movement into their routines, these healing arts have either classes or self-care practices. The workouts range from aerobic, for conditioning lungs and heart, to gentle range-of-motion movements, for flexibility.

BIOCHEMISTRY
❑ Aromatherapy
❑ Ayurveda
❑ Herbal Medicine
❑ Nutrition
❑ Polarity
❑ Traditional Chinese Medicine

These perspectives incorporate the use of food, herbs, and essences—a kind of better living through natural chemistry. Biochemical or energetic properties are ingested, inhaled, or absorbed through the skin. Many healing arts systems have nutritional philosophies as part of health-building.

MIND-BODY LINK

☐ Alexander Technique
☐ Autogenic Training and Therapy
☐ Bioenergetics and Body-Oriented Psychotherapies
☐ Biofeedback
☐ Feldenkrais Method
☐ Hypnosis and Hypnotherapy
☐ Past Life Therapy
☐ Relaxation Techniques
☐ Shamanism
☐ Tragerwork

While most healing arts recognize the body-mind continuum, these health care choices specifically access the body through the mind. They use techniques with psychoemotional effects, emphasize a learning process and/or aim to reeducate the brain. Some of the above practices can be attractive to intellectuals or people comfortable with imagery, verbalization, dialogue, or the discipline of set routines. However, a tendency to "stay in one's head" will reduce their effectiveness.

INTEGRATIVES

☐ Ayurveda
☐ Bioenergetics and Body-Oriented Psychotherapies
☐ Feldenkrais Method
☐ Iridology
☐ Martial Arts
☐ Rosen Method
☐ Yoga

Joseph Heller, creator of Hellerwork, proposes a category of bodywork he calls "integrative." He sees certain traditions trying to address more of the human being than just the physical. They use techniques that affect the mind, body mechanics, and energy. These are the arts that developed from a wider or more holistic sense of people and the healing process.

Jeffrey Low, who has created his own approach to bodywork called Neuro-Muscular Motivation, divides the body therapy continuum into relaxation, stimulation and manipulation segments. He describes the systems in the stimulation group as seeking to stimulate the body's own healing mechanism through the neuromuscular system, producing both mental and physical changes. There is no superimposed picture of an ideal body. Clients set the pace and depth of change. The goal is to maximize an individual's particular potential, whatever it may be at the time.

My view of the integrative arts incorporates both Heller's and Low's points of view, but goes a bit beyond. For instance, I include Iridology because it has developed a psychological component and usually includes herbal and/or nutritional counseling to effect body mechanics biochemically.

I'm not saying that these arts cover every health issue. Remember, "holistic" is an intent, a way of relating to a client, and a perspective on general health or on a particular condition and health. It is a capacity to see and understand, a way of approaching one's own life, work, and relationships, and not necessarily a scope of practice. If the practitioner has a holistic attitude, then the practice can be holistic, whether the scope of the technique is limited or broad. These arts attempt to integrate more aspects of the human experience within the scope of their approach and techniques.

Using Different Arts to Peel the Onion

Peeling the onion is a popular metaphor for journeying through self-knowledge. You strip back layer upon layer to get deeper, to approach the center. Pursuing health can be a similar process. Different healing arts are suited for different layers of your personal onion.

What begins as a weight issue can lead to dealing with food allergies and addictions. Bringing the allergies under control may include confronting the underlying emotional issues that fueled the food abuse that led to the allergies. Self-help groups and psychotherapy may help illuminate dysfunctional family issues that trained one as a child to turn to food for comfort. Healing childhood hurts and misconceptions may lead to learning less defensive behavior and more self-esteem.

Self-esteem and feelings of self-confidence can motivate and energize one to take up better health care habits, such as regular exercise, relaxation, and eating good food with good friends. Yoga classes, autogenic training, or Ayurvedic counseling can offer further self-regulation tools.

Rebirth of a healthy social life can bring better relationship skills and a better ability to maintain intimacy. Deeper and more meaningful contact with people not only satisfies the soul, it may also strengthen the immune system. The body increases its efficiency in metabolizing and cleansing itself of food. Colonics might help, too.

Body shape and feeling continue to change, aided by one of the soft tissue bodyworks or Rosen Method sessions. A massage becomes part of taking care of oneself and feeling good. The story can go on and on, spiraling upward to greater health and more satisfying experiences in life.

Spiraling Through the Layers of Your Onion

You can put together your own process using any of the tools in this book—or others that you may discover on your explorations. A spiral can also be a metaphor for movement through the complementary medicines, choosing different modalities as tools at different times or for different issues. Create your own spiral toward a general or specific health goal.

Be responsive to your inner voice and consider carefully any intellectual or emotional reaction you have to what you read in this book. Build partnerships with the practitioners you choose to consult. Discuss where your journey may lead you next as you peel your own onion.

You can concentrate on one healing art, going deeper and deeper into your own process with it. Or you can explore several arts within a family of healing arts. You can listen to your body or to an inner sense of what issue or aspect of yourself needs attention and look for a healing art that can help you address it.

There is no right way to do it, no one right goal or level of accomplishment in health. There is no set program of healing arts that will lead you to where you want to be.

Health and healing are dynamic, living processes. Every day is an opportunity to learn and appreciate who you are, to make choices about how to live your life and your health. The process, the journey, is unique to every individual, involving different genetic heritages, life incidents and decisions, and different health challenges, diseases, or wounds. Different people respond to different healers and healing arts; thus, the paths to health will also be unique.

The spiral captures the constant flow between opposite poles and a progression through time and space. It is an expression of the growth that can come from relapse, recuperation, and regeneration—and the movement toward ever-increasing awareness of our wholeness as living beings.

The Healing Arts

Acupressure

 ## What Is Acupressure?

Acupressure is a generic term encompassing any number of massage techniques that use manual pressure to stimulate energy points on the body. The masseur or masseuse applies light to medium pressure with fingers or hands—and sometimes elbows, knees, or feet—to the same points used in acupuncture. Many varieties of acupressure have developed over time. Some of the most well-known systems practiced in the West include:

Shiatsu: literally, finger (*shi*) pressure (*atsu*); a rhythmic series of finger pressures over the entire body along energetic meridians, or pathways, that also includes stretching and tapping. Points are held only 3 to 5 seconds. This treatment can be stimulating as well as relaxing.

Jin Shin: a pattern of gentle, prolonged point-holding of key acupuncture points on selected meridians and channels. Points are held for 1 to 5 minutes. Treatments are done in a meditative state to balance energy and body systems.

Do-In: a form of self-acupuncture massage of muscles and points that also includes movement, stretching, and breathing exercises.

Acu-Yoga: a series of yogic postures and stretches involving the whole body, that activate the points and meridian channels of acupressure.

Tui Na: Chinese massage that stimulates the acupressure points using a wide variety of hand movements.

Acupressure First Aid: a symptomatic approach using specific points for temporary relief of common conditions.

History and Development of Acupressure

Acupressure developed out of the human instinct to hold or massage parts of the body when they hurt. For example, we put our hands to our heads to clear our thoughts or massage headaches, or we hold our lower backs when they ache. These are all forms of unconscious self-acupressure.

Chinese Taoist monks began to formalize observations of this self-healing instinct over 5,000 years ago into a system called *Tao-Yinn* (*Tao*, "the way," and *Yinn*, meaning a gentle approach). It was both a therapy to cure specific complaints and a general health maintenance system. *Tao-Yinn* has come down to us as *Do-In*, the art of rejuvenation through self-massage.

Eventually, the Chinese added a system of diagnosis and treatment for a more complete medical approach.

Traditional Chinese Medicine traces its roots to these ancient philosophies and practices, together with centuries of observation and experimentation with energy theory and points. Chinese medical theory involves acupressure, acupuncture, moxibustion (using heat on acupuncture points), and herbology.

About 1,000 years ago, Chinese medicine arrived in Japan and was combined with Chinese massage (*amma*) techniques, the Japanese adding acupuncture points to their manual therapy. Eventually, the popular *shiatsu* emerged. Today it is authorized as a health treatment by the Japanese Ministry of Health and Welfare.

Shiatsu in Japan is an accepted medical treatment practiced by professionals with extensive training in diagnostic skills and *tsubo* (point) therapy. The shiatsu introduced in the West is mainly practiced for "home remedy" applications.

In the early 1900s, a Japanese philosopher named Jiro Murai developed another system of acupressure from his study of ancient literature and his 50 years of personal experimentation. He taught his *Jin Shin Jyutsu* or *Jitsu* to a Japanese-American woman who traveled to Japan after World War II to learn Japanese. Mary Ino Burmeister brought it back to America in the '50s, and she is the only teacher of this particular form. However, one of her students, Iona Teeguardan, developed a derivative form called *Jin Shin Do* that is now taught by training centers around the country. A student of Teeguardan, Michael Reed Gach, has created another form of self-acupressure, called Acu-

Yoga, that combines the techniques and benefits of yoga and acupressure.

Today, *jin shin* has blossomed into several individualized forms, some of which have been trademarked or incorporated. You can recognize them by the presence of a third word after *jin shin* in the marketing materials for treatments and classes. While it struck me at first that this was a particularly American kind of commercialization of the healing arts business, it really points to a deeper truth. Good teachers add something of themselves to whatever form they study and practice. Through experience, insight, and the occasional blending of other healing techniques into their treatment styles, gifted healers break out of the formula of the original style and create an expression of their own visions.

How Does Acupressure Work?

The technique's purpose is to stimulate the body's own recuperative powers. The giver of the acupressure massage holds or presses various points on the body or musculature to stimulate the body's electromagnetic energy. The stimulation removes energy blockages and fatigue by diffusing the lactic acid and carbon monoxide that accumulates in muscle tissue. This accumulation causes stiffness throughout the body and stagnation of the blood. Stiffness in the muscles puts abnormal pressure on nerves, and blood and lymph vessels that, in turn, affect both skeletal systems and internal organ functioning. Holding a leg cramp or kneading a sore back muscle can work the points that relieve the pain-producing symptoms and help restore muscle flexibility.

Electromagnetic energy is called by different names in different cultures—*chi* in China, *ki* in Japan, *prana* in India, and "the Force" in the movie *Star Wars*. It is considered the motivating life force common to all living things. Chinese medicine sees this vital force circulating throughout the body along specific pathways, called "meridians." The meridians, which are the same on both sides of the body, are our body's energy highway system. Energy flows up the front pathways and down the back ones. The meridians, in turn, flow from one into another, forming one continuous pathway on each side of the body.

In most people, when all pathways are open and energy flow is unhindered by muscle tension or other subtle blockages, the body's energy can be balanced. Balance brings good health, vitality, and a sense of well-being. When any of these pathways is blocked, proper application of finger pressure can loosen muscular tension, send the blood circulating, and stimulate or balance the flow of energy.

What Happens in an Acupressure Session?

While the specific techniques of acupressure differ, the goals are the same: to balance the flow of energy in the body, stimulating its own recuperative abilities. What changes from style to style (or even from practitioner to practitioner) is the different patterns of point holding, the number of points held, the length of time each point is pressed or held, the pressure used, and the technique of applying that pressure.

Regardless of the style, the first step for the acupressurist is to make an assessment. She may ask about your medical history and discuss with you what you are feeling or experiencing in your life at the moment and what kind of session might be most appropriate at this time. The practitioner may also use any one of the several traditional assessment techniques associated with acupressure, such as pulse diagnosis or face reading, an examination for signs of tension or disease, such as puffiness or dark circles around the eyes. Or she may examine the tongue or skin for indications of the condition of the internal energy flow. This is the time to mention symptoms, past or present injuries or operations, whether you are pregnant or have a skin condition, and any prescriptions you take or precautions from your doctor.

Acupressure can be performed while you are sitting in a chair or on a stool, or lying on a padded table or on carpeted floor. It can be done almost anywhere. Practitioners even give 15-minute sessions to office workers at their desks in downtown San Francisco. A quiet, relaxing atmosphere is most desirable, however.

Once the acupresssurist begins to hold or press points, you will soon notice a change in your breathing. Your normally shallow breath will slow down and deepen. Thoughts about what is happening in your life often fade as you turn your attention to the new body sensations. Focusing on the flow of your breath is part of the relaxation process and deepens the effect of the session. Don't talk. Let each deep breath out in a slow and conscious way, and notice muscles releasing their tension throughout your body. The practitioner should also breathe in slow, rhythmic, deeply felt breaths for acupressure to be most effective.

An acupressure treatment usually has two or three stages. First there is a general energy balancing, followed by specific attention to the blocked meridians that are at the root of the imbalance. Finally, many practitioners add some sort of a closing technique to bring the session to a gentle conclusion.

In a shiatsu session for the back, the practitioner will first stretch the back muscles by pushing up at the shoulders and down toward the feet at the small of the back. She will then slowly bend the legs toward the buttocks and squeeze the muscles along the sides of the torso before actually starting to apply pressure up the meridian points along the back.

In jin shin, the practitioner typically takes a pulse reading to determine how energy is flowing through the meridians, and then chooses specific points or a particular channel to use to establish overall balance. Once the body's energy is more balanced, the masseuse can focus on specific complaints, which usually stem from the key energy blockages. Treatment is usually given with the receiver lying on her back, fully clothed, and the practitioner and client are in a meditative state. The jin shin session ends with a neck and shoulder release.

Many practitioners create their own closing techniques to "seal" the energy balancing and/or to bring the client's awareness back to the everyday world. Sessions can be so deeply relaxing that you may fall into a sleeplike state and wake up somewhat disoriented or unsure of your movements for a few minutes. It is a good idea to lie on the table and appreciate the way your body has relaxed. Or, have the acupressurist grasp your feet or toes until you feel more awake.

Applications and Cautions

Acupressure is effective as a health maintenance system with regular, periodic sessions (once a week or once a month, for example) to reduce stress, increase circulation, and "tune up" your energy. You can choose acupressure to support other treatments or to give temporary relief for both chronic and functional ailments such as back pain, hypoglycemia, migraines, and cramps. It has first aid applications for traumatic conditions such as sprains, contusions, fractures, and vomiting. Individuals with internal diseases such as the common cold, ulcers, rheumatoid arthritis, paralysis, and gastrointestinal disorders can also benefit from acupressure. There are specific acupressure points to relieve common ailments such as asthma, constipation, insomnia, nosebleeds, sciatica, bedwetting, dizziness, fatigue, sore throat, and impotence.

Exercise caution if you are pregnant, have a skin condition, or an acute infectious disease. Acupressure experts do not recommend working in areas of tumor, especially malignant tumors, when there is danger of hemorrhaging.

Finally, some people may have a certain energy meridian assessed as "deficient." Whether by genetics, environment, or hard living, these channels routinely lack energy. They can be "balanced" into fullness by finger pressure. But acupressure is not a panacea. Diet and other lifestyle changes may be recommended or medical treatment required.

READ MORE ABOUT IT

ACUPRESSURE

The Joy of Feeling: Bodymind Acupressure
by Iona Marsaa Teeguarden
(Tokyo: Japan Publications, 1987)

Shiatsu Therapy
by Toru Namikoshi
(Tokyo: Japan Publications, 1974)

The Bum Back Book
by Michael Reed Gach
(Berkeley: Acu Press, 1983)

Acupressure Way of Health: Jin Shin Do
by Iona Teeguarden
(Tokyo: Japan Publications, 1978)

Chinese Massage Therapy: A Handbook of Therapeutic Massage
compiled by the Anhui Medical School Hospital, China
(Boulder, CO: Shambala, 1983)
(Tokyo: Japan Publications, 1981)

RESOURCES

American Shiatsu Association
P. O. Box 718
Jamaica Plain, MA 02130
(617) 236-2286
❏ information
❏ referrals and directory
❏ newsletter
❏ classes
❏ certification
❏ networking
❏ speakers
❏ convention

Acupressure Institute
1533 Shattuck Avenue
Berkeley, CA 94709
(415) 845-1059
❏ information
❏ referrals
❏ classes
❏ publications
❏ products
❏ training and certification

Jin Shin Do Foundation
P.O. Box 1097
Felton, CA 95018
(408) 338-9454
❏ information
❏ training and certification
❏ publications
❏ practitioners

Acupuncture and Traditional Chinese Medicine

What is Acupuncture and Traditional Chinese Medicine?

Acupuncture is one part of an ancient Oriental medical system developed in China. This therapy stimulates points on the body's surface to effect the physiological functioning of the whole body or specific parts. Points are stimulated by insertion of very fine needles, application of heat produced by burning an herb (mugwort)—called *moxabustion*—or application of pressure such as massage or acupressure.

Acupuncture is the most commonly known aspect of Traditional Chinese Medicine (TCM), a philosophy of nature that evolved into a complex system of examination and diagnosis of health and disease. TCM's courses of treatment can include herbal preparations, food therapy, exercise, and massage as well.

Chinese medicine uses over 4,000 herbs, many of which act synergistically when combined into prescription teas. Sometimes a Chinese doctor tells a patient to avoid or to eat certain foods. Exercise and lifestyle are also effective in building or depleting the body's energetic life force, or *chi*.

T'ai Chi Ch'uan is the most widely known form of Chinese exercise. We commonly see pictures of people of all ages practicing this gentle martial art in the parks and parkways of Chinese cities. *Qi Gong* (or *Chi Gung*), which means "manipulation of vital energy," is another martial art or physical meditation practice. It uses posture, movement, and breathing to foster a state of intense concentration as part of the physical training. Qi Gong masters demonstrate by breaking bricks with their foreheads, like karate masters.

Traditional Chinese Medicine has many similarities with other traditional Oriental medical systems from which it evolved, such as Indian Ayurvedic medicine. All of these traditional medical principles pivot on theories of energy and elements. They use herbs, food, exercise, breathing, and massage in a holistic approach to health. However, acupuncture in its present form is unique to Chinese medicine.

Traditional Chinese Medicine is a preventive medicine. In earlier days, patients paid the doctor as long as they were well and stopped paying him when they got sick. Today, many practicing acupuncturists do not use the entire system of Traditional Chinese Medicine but focus their efforts increasingly on the relief of specific symptoms.

Acupuncture has its own highly developed body of knowledge. To be properly used, it has to be based on a comprehensive medical education. There are three types of acupuncture used today:

❑ Traditional Acupuncuture: a preventive medicine for creating and maintaining health, usually practiced in conjunction with the full range of TCM techniques. Traditional acupuncture practitioners have years of study and training in the subtleties of Chinese medical philosophy.

❑ Symptomatic or First Aid Acupuncture: a formula approach for temporary relief of pain or discomfort without necessarily diagnosing the cause. The famous "barefoot doctors" in rural China practice this kind of acupuncture.

❑ Anesthetic Acupuncture: the use of needles instead of, or in conjunction with, anesthesia during surgery. A technique pioneered in the 20th century by the Chinese, who integrated Western and traditional Chinese medicines, we Westerners discovered it after Nixon first visited China.

In a recent development, some doctors use a very weak electrical current to stimulate the needles in the acupuncture points, instead of twisting the needles as in the traditional method.

History and Development of Acupuncture

One story has it that acupuncture was born from the observation that warriors wounded by arrows sometimes mysteriously recovered from chronic diseases unrelated to the areas of their wounds. While other cultures may have observed this phenomenon as well and tried using stone chips, sticks, and thorns to scratch and poke the skin as part of a healing routine, it was the Chinese who systematized acupuncture. They wrote one of the first books on it, *The Yellow Emperor's Classic of Internal Medicine,* which is still a basic text with information as applicable today as it was thousands of years ago, when it was written.

Acupuncture and Chinese medicine spread to Japan in the 6th century but it wasn't until the 17th century that French Jesuit missionaries there brought it to the West. They gave it its modern name, *acupuncture,* from the Latin roots *acus* (needle) and *punctura* (puncture). Needling became a fad in France for a while, and then fell into disrepute. It was "rediscovered" in the 1930s after a French sinologist and diplomat, Souli de Morant, published a series of detailed descriptions of the ancient art and its beneficial effects on the body.

By World War II, western medicine had made some inroads into China. TCM had been the only medical resource for Communist leader Mao Tse-tung, and it proved effective in preventing serious illness from defeating the Red Army during his long, arduous fight to take over the country. Since it was hard to obtain and distribute Western pharmaceuticals after the revolution, Mao ordered the training of both traditional and modern doctors. These eventually became the legions of paramedical "barefoot doctors" who served rural China, where the majority of that country's population resides. Today, both Western and traditional medicines are practiced in China, often side by side.

In the meantime, the West fell upon acupuncture as a new cure and began to dissect it with all its scientific tools. Doctors in Germany, France, Italy, and Argentina formed study groups and performed scientific experiments to explain how it worked.

In the '70s, *New York Times* columnist James Reston wrote about his appendectomy, which was performed using acupuncture instead of a pharmaceutical anesthetic, and acupuncture exploded on the American medical scene. Some doctors were incredulous, while others clamored for training. Debate and speculation flared up in the medical journals. While there is still some controversy, it has since died down. Today, the USSR, North and South Korea, and Japan have active research programs in the physiology and application of acupuncture.

How Does Acupuncture Work?

The ancient Chinese believed that we are born with a finite amount of energy circulating in our bodies, called *chi* or *qi*. This energy is captured and circulates in our bodies through invisible channels called meridians. The *chi* flows from one meridian into the other, completing an energy cycle every 24 hours, a dynamic force that animates us and our lives.

The amount and quality of this "prenatal" life force is determined by heredity, but how we live our lives also influences our *chi*. We enhance our store of energy by taking care of ourselves; we add to our energy by eating the right foods, supporting it with proper exercise, and breathing clean air. Sound familiar?

Our *chi* can be depleted by inappropriate living habits. The Chinese see the stresses of life that lead to imbalance or disease as:

❑ the six excesses: wind, cold, heat, dampness, dryness, and fire (these relate to TCM's theory of elements and its diagnostic language)

❑ the seven moods: joy, anger, anxiety, obsession, fear, horror, and sorrow

❑ intemperance in eating and drinking

❑ too little or too much sexual activity

❑ too little or too much exercise or work (or, in this "new age," too much—or too little—contemplation)

Any of these stresses and excesses can block the flow of *chi* in different parts of the body, or in the meridians. Illness is an excess or deficiency in the elemental energies in the body, an energy imbalance. Death is the absence or total depletion of this energy.

Acupuncture stimulates points on the energy meridians to unblock stuck energy, speed it up if it is flowing too slowly, or slow it down if it is racing too fast. Inserting and manipulating needles in the energy points, or "needling," corrects the imbalances that affect the functioning of our internal organs, which, in turn, affect our health.

There have been many theories proposed to explain how and why acupuncture works, especially as an anesthetic. In 1975, research in Russia and America led to the discovery of endorphins and enkephalins—natural painkillers produced by the body. These biochemicals also relieve allergies and depression, promote healing, and restore body functioning. The runner's "second wind" is a similar biochemical narcotic that the body creates to kill the pain of marathon exertion and stress on muscles. Acupuncture has been found to increase significantly levels of endorphins and enkephalins in the body.

Among the other theories proposed are:

❏ Placebo Effect: like the sugar pills research subjects believe are medicines, simply believing that acupuncture is effective marshals the body's own healing mechanisms.

❏ Hypnosis: more mind over matter; the power of suggestion associated with hypnosis or its state of heightened awareness stimulates physiological changes.

❏ Body Electricity: we generate a bioelectricity that flows through the meridians accessible at acupuncture points. Needling changes this electrical flow. Kirlian photography, which shows the body's aura in pictures, for example, of a hand or fingertip, is cited as evidence of heightened energy flow after acupuncture treatment.

❏ Gate Theory: both Chinese medical theory and Western research propose that there are (different) neuropathway gates to the brain along the spinal cord. Anesthetic acupuncture is supposed to close those gates, blocking the pain message so we don't feel it.

Yin/Yang and the Five Elements

Chinese medical theory grew along with Taoism, a philosophy that sees humans as a microcosm of the macrocosm of the universe. Every smaller part contains within it some pattern of the larger whole. This means that a medical practitioner can find out what is going on in the whole body by analyzing a part of the body, such as the hands, face, or feet.

Everything in the universe is made of the Five Elements— wood, fire, earth, water, and metal/air. And everything is governed by the opposite yet complementary forces of *yin* and *yang*.

The Chinese classify all things as *predominantly* yin or yang. Everything contains the seed of its opposite, as symbolized in the yin/yang sign. Yin is nurturing, embodying the feminine; yang is motivating, or masculine. Yin and yang coexist in a fluctuating harmony, one flowing into the other as night into day into night.

Each individual has a certain unique balance of yin and yang. Disturb this basic harmony and illness results. For example, too much yang may cause a fever; too much yin, a chill. Our health is a reflection of our relationship to these universal energies and the natural elements of life.

The Five Elements form dynamic energetic relationships between parts of ourselves. The acupuncturist describes each meridian of the body by both an element and an energy. The heart is said to be yin and fire, the small intestines are yang and fire. Each element has corresponding characteristics: flavor, sound, color, smell, direction, etc.

These characteristics are used to diagnose and describe the condition of a patient. The TCM doctor asks questions, observes, and tests to determine whether there is too much or too little of an element or energy.

What Happens in a Session?

It took me years to try acupuncture. I have had enough blood drawn and IVs inserted in my life to hate the thought of needles. I thought it would hurt. Actually, it's not so bad.

These needles are *very thin*. Some people might feel a slight prick when the needle goes in or a tug when it connects with an energy channel. Sometimes a muscle feels tight if it tenses up during needling. Once the needles are in, it is easy to forget they are there unless you look or move around.

A session starts with a diagnosis or assessment of your symptoms or complaints. The practitioner has four basic techniques for examination: to look, listen, ask, and feel. The acupuncturist will look at the color of your face, the condition of your tongue, skin, eyes, fingernails, and hair. She may ask for a urine or stool sample to check its color. She may also listen to the quality of your voice, its volume and force, and to the sound of your breathing or gurgles in your abdomen.

Most important, the practitioner will ask questions. She may want to know about your appetite, your body fluid secretions, and your individual and family medical history.

Finally, she will take your pulse, a main method for determining the condition of your body-energy flow. This is similar to the pulse reading your doctor or nurse performs except the acupuncturist will check three places from each wrist and three depths of flow at each place. With the information gleaned from the interview and pulse reading, the doctor will determine your specific imbalance and the point or points that will intervene.

The depth of the practitioner's training and experience, as well as the kind of treatment you want, determines how well acupuncture is going to serve your purpose—and how many sessions you need. Is it a quick fix, a first aid bandage on your condition, or a longer-term goal of health building and maintenance that you wish?

The acupuncturist, if she is a traditional Chinese medical doctor, may employ more than just the needles. She may decide that moxibustion or, more likely, herbal therapy will alleviate your condition and build your *chi*. The Chinese medical college graduate is really an herbal doctor. Acupuncture is only one part of an overall training in philosophy and techniques.

Applications and Cautions

Acupuncture is an energy medicine. It works by changing the quality or flow of the life force that energizes our tissues and organs. It is better suited to deal with functional illnesses and imbalances, or acute conditions that do not require the emergency treatment in which Western medicine excels. Sticking in needles may slow the flow of blood circulation and help alleviate high blood pressure, but if my leg is cut deeply and bleeding, I want a Western doctor to sew it up!

When checking clinics or practitioners, make sure they use sterilized disposable needles, and that before inserting the needle, the practitioner swabs the puncture site with alcohol or another disinfectant.

Acupuncture can be effective for insomnia, simple headaches, asthma and allergies, infertility, arthritis, menstruation and menopause problems, depression, and anxiety. Acupuncture is recommended for chronic conditions that do not respond to other treatments, gastrointestinal ailments, and conditions related to inflammation and lack of motility in joints.

In addition to emergency situations, acupuncture should not be used to treat vaginal discharges or undiagnosed pain. Any of these may be symptoms of conditions requiring surgery or antibiotics. Pregnant women should avoid acupuncture except as an anesthetic during delivery. Stimulating energy flow can induce an abortion or premature labor. Acupuncture is not a good idea for any kind of infection or as treatment for cancer, which might be spread by the increased energy flow and circulation.

You may have to think about whether you feel comfortable being stuck with needles. Are you so sensitive that you will have an emotional reaction to treatment? I had to work through feelings of being invaded or attacked, probably built up during an intense illness recovery period that included the frequent taking of blood samples.

Finally, there are different styles and schools of thought in the world of acupuncture: the original Chinese, and an English offshoot. The difference is not so much in needling technique as in recognition of an emotional, spiritual dimension of illness and treatment. Dr. Laurie M. Trujillo discovered she prefers acupuncturists trained in the Worsley, or English, tradition.

"It's the cultural difference," she says. "The Chinese doctor comes in, takes your pulse, inserts needles, and leaves without much explanation. I like someone who will discuss the diagnosis with me and give me feedback about the factors in my life that are contributing to my current state of health."

Trujillo made regular appointments to maintain an energy balance while in medical school at the University of California at San Francisco. She looked for a new acupuncturist to help her cope with even more grueling hours when she moved to Los Angeles to intern at UCLA Hospital. "I appreciate a practitioner who takes an ancient Eastern tradition, such as Chinese Medicine, and places it within a Western cultural context."

The English school not only recognizes the energetic relationships between meridians but also theorizes psychoemotional correspondences for each meridian-organ system. For example, they believe that experiencing grief may cause the lung meridian to become blocked. They may be right. After each TCM treatment for a lung imbalance, I would feel sad and cry a little. The mucus collected in my lungs, I reasoned, could be regarded as the sadness the treatment helped stimulate for release. The Chinese-born and trained acupuncturist seemed uninterested in my observations and questions about this. He said it was more a matter of my energy meridians being "a little mixed up." His American apprentices, more familiar with the English interpretations and California ways, responded to my need to discuss the idea. A Worsley practitioner will take great care to help a client work through an intense emotional response.

If you are looking for "bedside manner" to deal with a feeling or memory that the needling may bring up, consider the background of the acupuncturist. Ask during the initial interview about emotional side effects of treatment. Choose a practitioner who is willing to remain and talk with you during the 30 to 45 minutes that needles are left in, or to arrange for additional counseling.

READ MORE ABOUT IT

ACUPUNCTURE AND TRADITIONAL CHINESE MEDICINE

Staying Healthy With the Seasons
by Elson M. Haas, M.D.
(Millbrae, CA: Celestial Arts, 1981)

The Web that Has No Weaver: Understanding Chinese Medicine
by Ted J. Kaptchuk, O.M.D.
(New York: Congdon & Weed, 1983)

A Layman's Guide to Acupuncture
by Yoshio Manaka, M.D. and Ian A. Urquhart, Ph.D.
(New York: John Weatherhill, 1972/1980)

The Complete Book of Acupuncture
by Dr. Stephan Thomas Chang
(Millbrae, CA: Celestial Arts, 1976)

Clinical Acupuncture: A Practical Japanese Approach
by Katsusuke Serizawa, M.D.
(Tokyo: Japan Publications, 1988)

Chinese Medicine: Its History, Philosophy and Practice
by Manfred Porkert, M.D. with Dr. Christian Ullman
(New York: William Morris, 1982)

Encounters with Qi: Exploring Chinese Medicine
by David Eisenberg, M.D. with Thomas Lee Wright
(New York: W.W. Norton, 1985)

RESOURCES

American College of Traditional Chinese Medicine
455 Arkansas Street
San Francisco, CA 94107
(415) 282-7600
❏ information
❏ referrals
❏ training and certification
❏ publications
❏ speakers
❏ conference
❏ research

New England School of Acupuncture
30 Common Street
Watertown, MA 02172
(617) 926-1788
❏ information
❏ clinic
❏ training and certification
❏ speakers
❏ research
❏ seminars

Traditional Acupuncture Institute
American City Building, Suite 108
Columbia, MD 21044
(301) 596-3675
❏ clinic
❏ training
❏ publications
❏ speakers
❏ referrals

The Alexander Technique

What Is the Alexander Technique?

The Alexander Technique is a method of reeducating the body and mind to overcome poor habits of posture and movement and to reduce physical and mental tension. It is given as a series of lessons under the guidance of an Alexander teacher, during which a new way of organizing neuromuscular functioning to regain the natural use of one's body is explored.

History and Development of the Alexander Technique

The Technique was created by an Australian actor, Fredrick Matthias Alexander. Born in Tasmania in 1869, F.M. Alexander recited Shakespeare and poetry for a living. Concerned with a habitual loss of voice when he worked, he began to observe himself in a mirror to see what happened when he spoke. He noticed that when he started to speak —or just *thought* about speaking—he would pull his head back and tighten his throat.

Watching in a special three-way mirror, he studied his posture, movement, and balance. He discovered that his usual poor posture felt normal and the new posture, which reduced stress on his throat, felt strange. Practicing his new regime of speaking without pulling his head back, he soon felt healthier, more clear-headed, and more self-confident. His hoarseness disappeared and never returned. He eventually spent nine years studying himself and creating the Alexander Technique.

Alexander began to observe and work with others. He noticed they also had learned unnatural postures and inhibited movements: necks sunk into torsos, backs humped, or vertebrae contracted. He developed a method for retraining the body and forming good habits of posture and movement.

His discovery that people shorten their necks, a startle reflex pattern, led to a cornerstone of his theory, the concept of Primary Control. That is, there is a dynamic relationship of the head, neck, and back or torso that promotes maximum lengthening of the spine and facilitates movement throughout the body.

In 1904 Alexander moved to London and, slowly, his work gained recognition. In 1932, he published *The Use of Self*, which stimulated further interest in growth of the technique's popularity and acceptance. He toured and taught in England and America, leaving his younger brother, R.A. Alexander, to head the U.S. branch of the work. Studies of his methods were made by an American professor, Frank Pierce Jones, and an English doctor, Wilfred Barlow. Jones used multiple-image photography and X rays to observe the difference between habitual movement and movement guided by the Alexander Technique, while Barlow studied the connection between the "misuse of the body," as seen by Alexander, and medical disorders such as rheumatism, arthritis, back pain, hypertension, and spastic colon. Jones's and Barlow's findings supported the Technique's acceptance by some portion of the scientific and medical communities.

Alexander's most famous clients included Aldous Huxley, George Bernard Shaw, and Archbishop William Temple. Huxley endorsed the Alexander Technique in his book *Ends and Means*. The American educator John Dewey (creator of the Dewey Decimal System) reported improvement in his vision and breathing and considered the Technique a demonstration of the unity of mind and body. He wrote the foreword to Alexander's American edition of *Man's Supreme Inheritance*. Alexander died in 1955 in London, and today the work is carried out by the members of the Society of Teachers of the Alexander Technique. There are major schools in Chicago and San Francisco, throughout Europe, in Australia, and Israel.

How Does the Alexander Technique Work?

Alexander conceived the technique as a series of lessons in which the teacher, often using her hands, guides the pupil to experience his innate posture, movement, and balance. The focuses of the rediscovery process are the neck and head and their relationships to the rest of the body. The body's natural balance is lost in response to stress. To regain it, the pupil learns to change how he "uses" his body, increasing his daily awareness of posture and movement. This use, in turn, affects body functioning.

Frank Pierce Jones outlined three Technique hypotheses in his book *Body Awareness in Action*. First, our response to gravity, our effort to hold ourselves erect, is a basic organizing mechanism in life. Second, the pressures of modern life interfere with the fluidity and balance of this response. Third, becoming aware of this interference gives us the opportunity to inhibit the poor habits and integrate new ones.

We react to gravity and the stresses of modern life with learned stress responses—poor posture and inhibited movements. Two examples are pulling the neck down into the shoulder when startled or threatened and arching the back and puffing out the chest to bluff through difficult situations. Contractions and distortions in one part of the body can affect other parts, creating both physical and mental tension along with related emotional stress.

Conscious awareness of a shortened neck or hunched shoulders, and their effects on physical health and comfort, can inspire the pupil to change poor posture and movement habits. The Alexander Technique lessons help restore neuromuscular coordination as old, inhibiting patterns are replaced with freer, more flexible movement. The lessons show pupils how to use muscles the way they were originally designed to work.

Muscles contain nerves deeply imbedded in their long fibers. These spindle nerves send feedback to the brain, controlling muscle relaxation and contraction. Muscles act as shock absorbers in response to stimuli as we walk, jump, turn, and stop. Excessively or chronically contracted muscles, such as the shortened neck, inhibit muscle spindle nerves firing messages back to the brain. The muscles lose the response signals to keep fluid, be responsive, and absorb impact.

Pupils learn kinesthetic awareness skills—that is, awareness of body position, action, and movement—and use them to distinguish between poor and fluid movements. Jones explained that the Alexander lessons give pupils an immediate "aha" experience of performing a habitual act—walking, talking, breathing, handling objects—in a nonhabitual way.

Results take practice, practice, practice. Lessons are just the beginning, the first guided step in a process. The Technique is a discipline the pupils continue on their own. Further lessons are checks on the practice and serve as inspiration for deeper changes and improvement in body-mind functioning.

What Happens in an Alexander Technique Lesson

My first lesson was in a musty old vaulted classroom at Pomona College. I felt small when I walked into the room; much taller and lighter when I left. The teacher may start by having you stand or sit in a chair to observe how you hold yourself. My teacher had me get up from the chair a few times before "guiding my head" into a more natural, but less familiar balance. Gently pressing at the occipitals (the knobs at the base of the head), she gave me a new awareness of how my head felt on my neck, and how both felt in relation to my spine. She showed me how my normal (habitual) reflex was to pull my head back and my chin up when I prepared to stand, leading with my chin. "Is that how you go through your life—leading with your chin?" she asked.

Discovering that I respond to imagery, she suggested a mental picture of a very strong golden string attached to the crown of my head. With her help, I used that golden string to free myself from the sense that gravity was holding me down and to move up out of the chair. It was amazing, the difference in how I felt—lighter, more flexible, at ease with sitting and moving. Twelve years later, as I sit writing this, I remember the image of the golden string and feel myself recapturing that first lesson. It helps tremendously when I sit for hours at the computer.

In another lesson, she had me lie on a table on my back with my head resting on books. She had to stack several volumes before I could say the position felt comfortable since my neck was so habitually curved forward (more leading with my chin). She pointed out how I arched my back, holding myself up from the table. She told me to let the table support me. We talked about feelings of trust. She also drew my attention to a different sense of my body when my neck and head were in better balance. I felt poised when my neck was released, dropped back, and lengthened.

The key to the lessons is learning a new repertoire of posture and movement. The teacher calls attention to certain ways of holding, how we interfere with our innate ease of movement. You learn certain images or ideas which imprint the instructions and a kinesthetic memory of alignment. Those words and images become useful triggers for correcting poor habits of posture or movement on your own, as you continue to practice, practice, practice.

Applications and Cautions

In 1973, Nikolas Tinbergen devoted part of his acceptance speech for the Nobel Prize in Physiology and Medicine to an account of the Alexander Technique. He credited his and his family's "achievement of primary control" with alleviating high blood pressure and improving breathing, sleep habits, overall cheerfulness, mental alertness, and skill in playing a stringed instrument.

Recommendations and claims of improvement for the use of the Alexander Technique seem to fall into four categories:

❑ Chronic Conditions: therapy for backaches, TMJ (a painful jaw condition), stiff neck, asthma, headaches, depression, ulcers, spastic colon.

❑ Skill Development: relaxation techniques for use during physically active moments; prevention of tennis elbow; or improvement of sprinting performance.

❑ Performing Arts: economy of movement for dancers; breathing, voice, presence, and carriage for actors; holding instruments to prevent soreness or enhance expression for musicians.

❑ Personal Transformation: the Technique as a discipline for self-help, self-improvement; the "new age" awareness of self-responsibility and empowerment in developing the body as the temple of the soul.

The Alexander Technique can be a powerful tool for heightening self-knowledge and for changing habits; my teacher called it the development of conscious learning. I have friends who found it helped support their pursuit of other disciplines such as t'ai chi, yoga, and various kinds of meditation.

The challenge of the Alexander Technique is the practice. Results for this healing modality very much rest on the motivation and discipline of the client. The teacher can only teach so much. The real work is done on your own—in your awareness and practice of the new ways of carrying yourself. Lessons are only introductions, reminders, and feedback on your process and progress with the Technique.

READ MORE ABOUT IT

THE ALEXANDER TECHNIQUE

Body Learning: An Introduction to the Alexander Technique
by Michael Gelb
(New York: Delilah Books, 1981)

Body Awareness in Action
by Frank Pierce Jones
(New York: Schocken Books, 1976)

The Use of Self
by F. Matthias Alexander
(New York: E.P. Dutton, 1932; Centerline paperback, 1986)

F. Matthias Alexander: The Man and His Work
by Lulie Westfeldt
(Long Beach, CA: Centerline Press, 1984)

The Alexander Technique
by Wilfred Barlow
(New York: Alfred A. Knopf, 1973)

The Universal Constant in Living
by F. Matthias Alexander
(New York: E.P. Dutton, 1941; Centerline paperback, 1986)

RESOURCES

The American Guild of Teachers of the Alexander Technique
931 Elizabeth Street
San Francisco, CA 94114
(415) 550-7340
❏ information
❏ referrals
❏ classes
❏ training and certification
❏ speakers

North American Society of Teachers of the Alexander Technique
P.O. Box 806, Ansonia Station
New York, NY 10023-9998
(212) 866-5640
❑ information
❑ teacher list
❑ publications
❑ training

Aromatherapy

What Is Aromatherapy?

Aromatherapy employs aromatic essences extracted from wild or cultivated plants for beauty treatments or therapies similar to those used in herbal medicine. The essential oils are organic compounds that produce a wide range of therapeutic responses. Though usually administered by massage, in baths, and through inhalation, these oils may also be taken internally when prescribed by medical doctors.

History and Development of Essential Oil Therapies

Though not termed "aromatherapy" until the 1920s, the use of plant essences dates back at least to the time of the pharaohs. Egyptians used aromatic herbs, woods, and resins to mummify their cats and kings. Archaeologists found pots of scented unguents in King Tut's tomb. The antiseptic power of natural essences such as myrrh and cedarwood can arrest putrefaction.

The ancient Egyptians found uses for plant essences in their daily lives as well. Men of that time perfumed themselves by placing on their heads cones of solid animal fat mixed with aromatic oils, which would slowly melt over them during the day. And in at least one city, Tel-el-Amana, piles of aromatic plants were burned in public squares to purify the air.

Essential oil therapy practices, such as "smoking" a patient with incense, came down through history from the Greeks who studied Egyptian medicine. An Arab physician, Avicenna, is credited with refining the technique of distillation extraction, the most common form of obtaining a plant's essential oil.

As in Egypt, aromatic woods were burned in the streets of

69

Europe during the Great Plague. Aromatics were then the best known antiseptics, so hospitals were fumigated with incense, and scented candles burned in sickrooms. Medieval doctors tried every essence, from pine and sulphur to pepper and frankincense, to fight the Black Death.

In the seventeenth century, herbalists flourished, especially in England, and doctors used essential oils as a comprehensive part of their medicine. However, aromatherapy declined after the Renaissance as pharmacists and chemists developed the principles of modern chemistry.

Modern aromatherapy was born in France earlier this century with the research of Rene Maurice Gattefosse, a chemist in his family's perfume factory. Aware of the medicinal history of essential oils, he plunged his hand into a container of pure lavender oil after burning it in a laboratory explosion. His hand healed in hours with no sign of infection or scarring. This incident led him to develop the use of essential oils in dermatology. He published his findings in a scientific paper in 1928 titled "Aromatherapie." The name stuck.

Two modern proponents of aromatherapy, Marguerite Maury and Dr. Jean Valnet, brought aromatherapy to the attention of the medical world, as well as the health and beauty industries. Mme. Maury, a biochemist, and her husband, a homeopath, translated traditional aromatherapy practices into modern techniques. Her book, *The Secret of Life and Youth*, published in 1962, focused on cosmetology, emphasizing the rejuvenative properties of essential oils.

Valnet, a medical doctor and former army surgeon, used essential oils to treat severe burns and other battle injuries. He later treated veterans in psychiatric hospitals with different aromatics. Many of these patients, who suffered psychoemotional effects from their war experiences, showed marked improvements after Valnet's therapy. Beginning his medical writings on aromatherapy in the 1960s, he published an English translation of his classic handbook, *The Practice of Aromatherapy*, in 1982.

Aromatherapy is mostly a medical and naturopathic domain in France. Pharmacies throughout Europe sell essential oils along with homeopathic remedies and allopathic (modern medical) drugs. Purchase of aromatherapy oils is reimbursed by French health insurance.

Today essential oils flavor foods, perfume cosmetics, and strengthen medicines. Some toothpastes contain clove oil; several inhalants and cough drops get their menthol from eucalyptus. In America and Britain, use of essential oils for home remedies grows in popularity, but aromatherapy is still considered a "fringe medicine."

However, the American Aromatherapy Association, which held its first convention in 1988, is working to improve that image. This professional group pledges to create quality standards and to increase public awareness of the benefits of aromatherapy.

How Does Aromatherapy Work?

Like many other traditional healing arts, we don't know *exactly* how aromatherapy works. Chemists have isolated separate fragrant molecules in the oil created in the chloroplasts of leaves. A Russian study found that evaporation of the essences acts as a defense mechanism. Various compounds act as pesticides, bactericides, and fungicides for the plant.

The oils are also regulators and messengers for some plants, a kind of hormonal response to help them adapt to a stressful environment. In fact, sage contains an estrogen. Native American women traditionally have used this herb to help regulate menstruation. Ginseng, known as a tonic and aphrodisiac, contains a compound similar to folliculin, an estrogen released during pregnancy.

But what do these fragrant materials do for, or to, us? We can begin to answer this by understanding that our sense of smell works on a subconscious level. Olfactory nerves connect to the brain's limbic system, which also regulates sensory motor activities and affects sexual urges and behavioral mechanisms. This confluence of neurological wiring means that smell can affect emotional behavior. The perfume industry grasped this early and ever since has used sex to sell its products.

Olfactory nerves affect memory, also. A French psychoanalyst, Andre Virel, uses fragrances in his practice to bring out patients' hidden memories. Like smelling salts, different odors wake up the brain, evoking images and feelings associated with each smell. A study at Warrick University in England found that simply smelling a beach can be relaxing. Students in a lab experiment sniffed ozone and such coastline odors as seaweed and rotting clams. Relaxation responses in some students increased up to 17 percent.

When absorbed by the skin, inhaled, or ingested, essential

oils are transported throughout the body to affect various organ functions. For example, oils can act as sedatives or stimulants, carminatives (agents that expel intestinal gas), and digestive aids, or cause numerous other real physiological effects in the body. Most contemporary aromatherapy literature highlights the symptomatic uses. But like aspirin, used for decades before its exact biochemical properties were discerned, most oils produce benefits that are time-tested even while their mechanisms are not completely explained.

Many proponents give a metaphysical explanation for how aromatherapy works. Like flower essences and herbal remedies, essential oils, practitioners say, contain the vital energy of the plant. Each plant part, even its roots and resin, carries an imprint or pattern of its personality and spirit. The essence captures the most ethereal and subtle part of the plant. Some say that the essential oil, therefore, can have even more profound effects on the mind and emotions than herbal medicine.

Applications and Cautions

Aromatherapy is used to treat physical ailments as well as to reap psychological or spiritual benefits. The oils are applied through several methods, especially massage, baths, skin preparations (salves), compresses, and steam inhalations.

Many of the recent books in English about aromatherapy describe the different physiological actions of various oils and applications for symptom relief. Some oils have a normalizing effect, acting to strengthen the body's own regulatory actions. Hyssop and garlic oils, for example, can be useful in treating both high and low blood pressure.

Aromatherapy has helped to combat wrinkles, acne, and other skin problems as well as to treat poor circulation, obesity, broken capillaries, rheumatism, sinusitis, and depression, anxiety, and stress.

Massage is the most effective way to introduce essential oils to the body. The stimulation and relaxation of the massage help the essences penetrate the skin. Circulating blood and relaxed muscles improve absorption and distribution of the oils' active ingredients. And just for pure enjoyment, nothing beats a soothing Swedish or Esalen massage scented with a favorite flower oil.

Aromatherapists, especially those who treat skin conditions

with therapeutic massage, may have their clients fast or modify their eating for several days to help improve the efficiency of the treatment. Healthy skin also helps. Acne and other skin disorders often indicate congestion in the skin and lymph glands, the medium of transmittal for the healing oils. Oils aid the body's own immune system to combat germs and impurities; so the clearer the field of battle, the better the chances of winning.

Another popular method of treatment is an aromatic bath. Baths can be tonic or sedative, relaxing or stimulating, aphrodisiacal, warming or cooling. Used to relieve muscular pain and skin conditions, they can also reduce the effects of stress. Hot water opens pores and helps the body absorb the oils more quickly. It also turns some of the oil into aromatic vapor, to be gently inhaled as you soak.

Take particular care with baths, however. Just a few drops of essence will do a lot for you in hot water. The oils spread out in a thin layer on the surface of the water, coating you as you enter the bath. Some of the stronger oils, such as basil, rosemary, and peppermint, may burn your skin a bit.

Also, match the temperature of the water to your purpose and oil. Hot baths are stimulating and strengthening (if kept short), and tepid baths are relaxing and sedative. A lavender bath can be soothing but if the water is too hot, it will counteract the oil's effects.

Foot baths suffice if you don't have a bathtub or are immobilized in some way. The soles of the feet readily absorb the oils. A foot bath after a little foot reflexology can be quite effective.

Take precautions when using essential oils for home remedies. Many of the stronger-scented oils may counteract homeopathic therapy. If under treatment, check with your homeopath before using any oils.

Aromatherapists have identified particular oils that can combat specific conditions. However, you may experience a negative reaction with some oils. Test an oil before diving into a hot bath or massaging it all over your body. I discovered a sensitivity to eucalyptus the hard way, giving myself a more excruciating headache than the one I tried to cure.

It is vital that you take great caution with the amount of oil you use. Some oils are poisonous except in the smallest amounts. Pennyroyal is one of several oils that can cause miscarriages. Marjoram, which can prevent spasms or convulsions, can be stupefying in high dosage. An overdose of saffron, a cerebral stimulant, can trigger convulsions, delirium, and even death.

Some books suggest ingesting a few drops of oil on a sugar cube or with honey in tea. This practice was developed in Europe where most of the aromatherapy practitioners are medical, homeopathic, or naturopathic doctors; I question this use in unmonitored home remedies.

Working with oils, you will discover that most are too strong to apply directly to the skin, much less to swallow. Take note. Sugar or honey will make the oil go down more easily. But the oil will still be as rough on the alimentary canal as it was on the skin, and the effects can be even more severe.

Under a doctor's care and direction, it may be safe to take oils internally. However, anything but external self-medication—compresses, massages, hot baths or salves—is unwise and risky.

I have been using aromatherapy to reduce stress, balance digestion, and indulge my senses ever since I read Robert Tisserand's *The Art of Aromatherapy*. Now my travel first aid kit always includes peppermint for stomach troubles, lavender for cuts and bites, sage or thyme for sinus headaches and colds, and rosemary to wake me up with a morning footbath or for a balancing bath at night.

READ MORE ABOUT IT

AROMATHERAPY

The Practice of Aromatherapy
by Jean Valnet, M.D.
(New York: Destiny Books, 1980)

The Art of Aromatherapy: The Healing and Beautifying Properties of the Essential Oils of Flowers and Herbs
by Robert B. Tisserand
(New York: Inner Traditions International, 1977)

Aromatherapy for Women
by Maggie Tisserand
(New York: Thorson Publications, 1985)

Aromatherapy: An A-Z
by Patricia Davis
(Essex, England: C. W. Daniel Company, 1988)

RESOURCES

American Aromatherapy Association
P.O.Box 1222
Fair Oaks, CA 95628
(916) 965-7546
❑ information
❑ referrals
❑ membership newsletter

Pacific Institute of Aromatherapy
P.O.Box 606
San Raphael CA 94915
(415) 459-3998
❑ information
❑ publications
❑ products

The Tisserand Aromatherapy Institute
3 Shirley Street
Hove, East Sussex, BN 3WJ
England
0273-772-479
❑ information
❑ publications

Autogenic Training and Therapy

What Is Autogenic Training?

Autogenic Training (AT) is a highly systematized series of attention-focusing exercises designed to generate a state of mind and body relaxation. The training is the foundation for Autogenic Therapy, a process especially applicable to psychosomatic disorders. Autogenics is a kind of self-hypnosis, and is used to gain deep relaxation and enhance one's recuperative and self-healing powers.

Autogenic means self-generated. AT's purpose is to give trainees the skills to put themselves in a relaxed state without depending on a trainer or guide. This state, akin to hypnosis or meditation, allows the body to release its own stress, muscle tension, and neuromuscular memories, the body's subconscious recollection of previous physical and emotional traumas. This relaxation and release frees the body to return to a homeostasis, or equilibrium.

History and Development of Autogenic Training

Autogenics grew out of research in the late 1880s at the Berlin Neuro Biological Institute. Brain physiologist Oskar Vogt noticed that some patients could put themselves into a self-hypnotic state. This state seemed to have positive effects on their recuperative processes. Vogt and his colleague, Korbinian Brodmann, began to experiment and develop self-hypnosis techniques and to report on the clinical value of their "prophylactic rest-autohypnosis" exercises. Done several times a day, patients experienced relief of such conditions as headaches and fatigue and tension due to stress.

Some years later, the report inspired Johannes Schultz, a Berlin psychiatrist and neurologist, to investigate the therapeutic potential of hypnosis. His interest was the self-directed nature of the autohypnosis exercises, which decreased the patient's dependency on the therapist. Schultz, along with his student Dr. Wolfgang Luthe and others, created the exercises that became Autogenic Therapy.

The difference between AT and hypnosis is the autogenic intent to induce experiences common to hypnotic states, but not the hypnotic state itself. The goal is to invoke the sensations, beginning with the warmth and heaviness of the extremities, experienced in hypnotic states. The experimenters above created six "standard exercises" to attain a warm abdomen, a cool forehead, and a passive, nonstriving attitude.

Menninger Foundation researchers Elmer and Alyce Green stumbled upon a book by Schultz and in 1966 began to investigate Autogenic Training using equipment and methodology that eventually developed into the biofeedback field (see Biofeedback). Their electronic equipment measured respiration, heart rate, galvanic skin response, blood flow, and hand temperature. The Greens called their marriage of biofeedback machines and AT "autogenic feedback training." Among their results was a system to relieve migraine headaches.

By the late '60s the popularity and further development of AT had spawned a six-volume summary of research and methodology, edited by Luthe. The international textbook compiled papers, clinical and experimental observations, and general information from members of the International Committee for the Coordination of Clinical Application and Teaching of Autogenic Therapy—ICAT for short. Autogenic Training was now a worldwide therapy method.

A full-fledged bridge between the bailiwicks of the medical world and the psychotherapeutic world, Autogenic Therapy continues to grow as a tool for individual healing and self-empowerment. Research and theoretical dialogue continue, addressing AT medical applications, psychotherapeutic approaches, and autogenic modifications, meditation, and neutralization techniques.

How Does Autogenic Therapy Work?

Autogenics, like other relaxation techniques, directs the individual to concentrate on bodily sensations and breathing. The six basic meditative exercises for Autogenic Training focus on:

❑ relaxing the neuromuscular system

❑ relaxing the vascular system

❑ regulating/adjusting the heart rate

❑ the breathing mechanism

❑ creating warmth in the abdomen

❑ cooling the forehead

For people who master the first set of exercises, there are three further techniques to use for continued release or relaxation. Autogenic meditation is a series of structured meditations designed to help you reach more deeply into your unconscious mind. The practitioner directs the trainee toward passive concentration on a visual, such as a color or an object, and then on an abstraction, such as happiness or justice. Then the trainee can move to personal feelings or an image of another person. Finally, at the deepest level, the exercise trains one to ask questions and receive answers from the one's own unconscious.

Autogenic modification is directed toward a specific organ or body part to promote functional changes in order to overcome such chronic conditions as allergies, diarrhea, weight difficulties, or behavioral problems. Clients use "intentional formulas" as affirmations to give the body information or a posthypnoticlike suggestion. For example, an affirmation for hay fever is "Pollen doesn't matter," to help the body stop overreacting to pollen.

Autogenic neutralization digs deep to uncover particularly introspective psychophysical blockages, using stream-of-consciousness verbalization to trigger more powerful or intense releases. While it's possible to attempt neutralization on your own, this technique is most effective under the guidance of a trainer.

Dr. Herbert Benson, author of *Relaxation Response*, asserts that profound relaxation turns off the chronic release of stress chemicals from the brain so the body can focus on normal self-healing. And like REM (rapid eye movements) and dreams during sleep, or muscle jerks during a deep bodywork session or in the isolation tank, AT facilitates spontaneous, normal discharges of energy.

What is clear about AT is that it can, with practice, help its users attain a profound state of relaxation. Deep relaxation, whether through AT, meditation, or sensory deprivation (flotation tank) can help promote homeostasis, the body's ability to determine and regain its own normal self-regulation.

Autogenics assumes a deep faith in the brain's (and body's) own ability to regulate itself. That is, the energy releases will be kept under control. The body will not unload these stored episodes faster or more intensely than the individual can handle. Like a typical healing crisis in most medical systems and healing arts, the release may be intense but not life threatening. With trainer guidance and trainee self-responsibility, the process can go as fast or slow, as far or deep, as the individual chooses.

What Happens in a Training Session?

AT is taught in a structured fashion; a trainer monitors the client's progress. The process begins with the therapist taking a detailed medical and psychological history. This acts as a guide so both the trainer and the client know what neuromuscular memories the process might release.

The trainee keeps a diary or log, noting feelings, images, or physical events that occur during training. The trainer judges whether and how soon the client can move to the next exercise. Clients practice the exercises for several minutes, three times a day. When applied to supporting treatment for a particular condition, it usually takes two to six months for the training to effect reversal of pathology. But one can begin to release neuromuscular imprints or reactions connected to repressed physical or emotional pain as soon as one masters a state of profound relaxation.

One example, from my experience, of the release of an unexpressed or stored trauma resulted from the broken elbow I suffered 10 years ago after slipping off a stool. I called my husband to take me to the hospital but it took an hour for him to get home. At the time, I acted very brave about the pain and very polite about the delay. I kept both the physical trauma and the unexpressed emotional upset of the incident bottled up inside, where they remained, waiting to be released.

In fact, when I learned to drop into the autogenic state, my elbow did begin to twitch and ache. Later, I watched as mild waves of anger and blustery tears came over me. The autogenic state helped me let go enough to allow my body to "unload" the pain, tears, anger, and memory of the initial injury. Hopefully, the energy it took to hold that pain in my elbow will now act instead to make it feel less fragile.

Applications and Cautions

While there is little well controlled research into AT's principles, clinical evidence suggests it is useful both as a primary and as a supportive technique for diverse medical conditions. These include gastritis, hypertension, asthma, diabetes mellitus, arthritis, sinus tachycardia (racing heart), premature ejaculation, and alcoholism. The Greens's application of autogenic biofeedback training to migraine headaches shows the technique's success in affecting blood vessel constriction and control of blood flow. Almost any psychosomatic illnesses and many anxiety- or stress-related conditions can be responsive to AT.

Autogenic therapists are developing further applications, especially in the areas of education, industry, and sports. These new autogenic techniques can, for example, help strengthen concentration and endurance abilities, and reduce anxiety.

Some of the cautions and limitations of autogenics are similar to those of other relaxation and meditation techniques. It probably will not work for people who cannot follow instructions, such as young children or schizophrenics, or for rebellious or unmotivated individuals.

Some medical needs may not be best served by the technique or may demand exclusion of certain exercises. Clients should have full medical examinations to determine that any pain is not due to angina or a brain tumor, for example. These are conditions requiring immediate medical treatment, not an autogenic discharge.

Certain exercises may result in adverse reactions when focused on an issue or area of pathology. Take care with conditions where anxiety about the process or the particular exercise could dangerously exacerbate an existing medical condition. A peptic ulcer patient or pregnant woman may want to skip the "solar plexus warming" exercise. Likewise, a heart patient should omit the heart rate exercise or use it under strict medical supervision.

Finally, mastering the autogenic exercises and attaining profoundly deep relaxation states may necessitate lower dosages of blood pressure medicine for hypertension patients or insulin for diabetics. If you are being treated for either of these conditions, alert your primary care provider to the potential effects of autogenics so she can monitor and adjust your medication promptly.

READ MORE ABOUT IT

AUTOGENIC TRAINING AND THERAPY

Autogenic Training: A Psychophysiologic Approach to Psychotherapy
by J. Schultz and W. Luthe
(New York: Grune and Stratton, 1959)

Autogenic Therapy
Volumes I–VI
edited by Wolfgang Luthe, M.D.
(New York: Grune and Stratton, 1969)

RESOURCES

International Committee for Autogenic Training
101 Harley Street
London, W1N 1DF
England

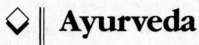

◇ Ayurveda

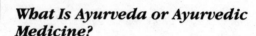

What Is Ayurveda or Ayurvedic Medicine?

Ayurveda is a traditional medicine from India incorporating medicinal, psychological, cultural, religious, and philosophical concepts. Sometimes called the "mother of all healing," Ayurveda means knowledge (*ayur*) of life (*veda*). Ayurvedic medicine is a practical "science of life," with principles for better health that can be applied to any individual's daily life.

Developed in India over the past 4,000 years, Ayurveda's eight main branches (or "limbs") of medicine are: pediatrics, gynecology, obstetrics, ophthalmology, geriatrics, otorhinolaryngology (ears, nose, throat), surgery, and general medicine. Each type of medicine is addressed in terms of the three *doshas* (bodily elements or "bioforces") and the patient's constitutional type.

History and Development of Ayurvedic Medicine

Ayurveda is based on the ancient wisdom of the *rishis*, holy wisemen who divined the principles of this science through religious introspection and meditation. It is mentioned in the *vedas*, the oldest sacred scriptures of India. Compilation and documentation of Ayurvedic knowledge is found as well in the *samhitas*, written 2,000 years ago.

Charak Samhita includes a comprehensive treatise elaborating on eight major branches of human health care, from psychology and toxicology to rejuvenation and virilization. *Sushrita Samhita*, written by a surgeon, details such procedures as plastic surgery, postmortem dissection, knitting bones together with nails, bloodletting to cure blood-borne disorders, and manipulating vital energy points (*marmas*), similar to acupuncture points.

That Ayurveda and Traditional Chinese Medicine (TCM) share similar concepts, such as energy points, pulse diagnosis, and herbal remedies, is no accident. Both spring from the same historical roots. Both cultures, for example, traced their origins to a mythological group of seven sages symbolized by the stars of the Big Dipper. Indian and Chinese cultures developed in proximity to each other, while the spread of Buddhism fostered even more interchange. Early Buddhist scholars in China were also Ayurveda practitioners.

Both Oriental medicines organize food, herbal remedies, and energies into five elements. The Chinese divide the world and its material into *yin* and *yang*; the Indians into three bioforces: *vata*, *pitta*, and *kapha* (usually translated as wind, fire, and mucus). Both Ayurveda and TCM use energetic concepts to characterize and explain all life experiences.

As Traditional Chinese Medicine grew in strength and organization, however, it eventually overshadowed Ayurveda in China. But Ayurveda continued to develop in India, despite invasions and conquerors who tried to subsume the local culture and wisdom.

Ayurveda is said to have used needles at one time, perhaps in connection with the *marmas*, but needle use died out early. It is possible that records of acupuncturelike practices were burned in the wars. Actually, Ayurvedic traditions have been better preserved in the medical tradition of the isolated Tibetans. Many scholars, in fact, are turning to Tibet to understand the origins of this medical philosophy.

Tibet, the crossroad between the two great countries and cultures of India and China, has integrated principles from both Ayurveda and TCM into its unique and somewhat esoteric Tibetan Medicine. Tibetan Medicine explains health in the same three bioforces as Ayurveda. It also uses pulse reading in diagnosis and herbs as medication. However, unlike TCM practitioners, Tibetan doctors take pulses at various points on the arms and fingers, not just at the wrist.

To early twentieth-century Westerners, Indian health practices seemed primarily to involve yoga and meditation. Indeed, these are important adjuncts to Ayurvedic medicine. Breathing and stretching exercises, developed over the centuries to quiet the mind and spirit and energize the body, are integral to the preventive health approach of Indian medical philosophy.

In the 1960s, yoga and meditation dawned on the American

consciousness as separate entities. Richard Hittleman's and Lilias's PBS series on Hatha yoga imported *asanas* (yoga poses or exercises) and *pranayama* (yoga breathing) into our living rooms. The Beatles, meanwhile, called the world's attention to Maharishi Mahesh Yogi. His gleeful laugh and promotion of Transcendental Meditation (TM) caught the imaginations of many. Hundreds of thousands of potentially stressed-out Americans have adopted one piece of the Ayurveda way of life—stopping to meditate at least once a day.

Today, the Maharishi is working to bring the rest of Ayurveda to America. Several "Maharishi Ayurveda Centers" dot the country from Boston to Los Angeles. They offer a capsulized version of Ayurveda practices. Health seekers can purchase beautifully packaged herbal remedies and condiments for balancing various constitutional disorders, sign up for detoxifying massages, and learn other stress-reducing and health-building techniques based on Ayurvedic principles.

Meanwhile, in Honesdale, Pennsylvania, the Himalayan Institute has been publishing books and offering health programs and retreats based on Ayurveda since the 1970s. Codirected by a Harvard-trained cardiologist, Dr. John Clark, and Dr. Rudolph Ballentine, the Institute focuses on stress reduction and chronic diseases. The Institute's simple, easy-to-understand books outline many aspects of lifestyle, health, and spiritual practices that spring from Ayurvedic traditions. Ballentine's 1978 tome, *Diet and Nutrition,* is a classic text on the body's inner workings, composition, digestion, absorption, and elimination of food.

The third major location for Ayurvedic study in the United States is the Ayurveda Institute and Wellness Center, in Santa Fe, New Mexico, headed by a prominent Indian doctor, Dr. Vasant Lad. It offers health management counseling, traditional detoxifying and cleansing treatments, and training for Ayurvedic consultants. Dr. Lad, a popular lecturer on Ayurveda throughout the country and Europe, was formerly a professor and director of clinical medicine at Poona University College of Ayurvedic Medicine in India.

How Does Ayurveda Work?

Ayurveda sees human beings as complex entities made up of unique combinations of elements called *doshas.* Santa Cruz Ayurveda consultants Ashwin and Dev Priya Hansen have referred to these *doshas* as "bioforces," interacting to create biological activities.

Vata produces movement (wind) in the body. *Pitta* is the force of heat (fire), such as digestion. *Kapha* is the bioforce for growth and structure, the elements of earth and water that create mucus. The common cold, for instance, is an overabundance of kapha.

The mixture of these bioforces creates our individual constitution, or *prakruti*. The heart of Ayurveda's view of human health and disease is its analysis of each individual's unique prakruti and ways of keeping these bioforces in balance for optimum health.

Good health, in Ayurvedic medicine, is a state of balance where one's body, mind, spirit, and environment are in harmony. This harmony is achieved through the observation of proper diet, exercise, and lifestyle habits; the practice of meditation; and the maintenance of psychological wellness, especially through the serenity that comes with self-acceptance and love.

Ayurveda rarely treats symptoms. It focuses on curing disease by removing the cause of the "dis-ease." Causes are transgressions against Nature's laws, crimes against inner wisdom. They include the excessive use of our senses, or the ignoring of the time cycles of the day, season, or our age. At the same time, Ayurveda keeps the body's immune system strong and able to combat everyday germs or to heal itself of chronic disorders.

Treatment goals include restoring energetic balance, strengthening the immune system, and helping the body take care of itself. Ayurveda heals with synergistic herbal remedies, body cleansing routines, yoga, meditation, and dietary changes.

Ayurvedic consultants analyze clients' constitutional makeup and help them improve their lifestyle habits to better suit their own particular constitutional needs. There are seven constitutional types, or different mixtures of the three *doshas*. Once you know your constitutional type, you can begin to work with your nutrition, exercise, and psychological needs, to pacify an aggravated bioforce and bolster another deficient one. You create your own individualized health maintenance system, based on your *prakruti*.

Diet, which is tied to the power of digestion, is a primary concern. There are foods that disturb one bioforce but enhance or pacify another. Each bioforce has its own dietetic needs. For instance, eating a light breakfast or fasting one day a week can benefit *kapha*-dominant types, as it helps clear out the overabundance of mucus. However, fasting can "lighten up" *Vata* types too much. *Vatas* are the nervous, on-the-go people. They usually need foods to help them stay calm and grounded.

However, a client is not tied to one list of foods or eating regimen. Ayurvedic consultants guide clients in choosing optimum eating routines based on the season of the year or their particular imbalances.

What Happens in a Session?

The initial consultation evaluates one's constitutional type and current state of elemental balance. *Prakruti* is determined by a complex system of analysis. The consultant starts with pulse reading, involving a sophisticated system of 12 positions on both arterial pulses at the wrists. The pulses are read to learn the mixture of the three bioforces in the client's constitution, and to recognize the balance or imbalance in the client's various organ functions.

After reading the pulses, the doctor or consultant is able to draw a picture of the client's *vikriti*, or general state of health. They feel for such things as pace, strength, depth, and pattern of movement. A pulse can be slow and steady, thready like a snake, or jumpy like a frog. Each portrait or metaphor helps to sketch a picture of the client's condition in terms of the three bioforces, *vata*, *pitta*, and *kapha*.

The client also answers a series of questions or fills out a survey of characteristics to help confirm the pulse reading analysis. The Ayurvedic consultant may also do a visual analysis, including tongue, fingernails, eyes, urine and feces, the face and skin, and observe voice quality and breath odor. The external features give indications of internal conditions. A white tongue with teeth marks around the edge, for example, shows low digestive bioforce.

Once the analysis is complete, the counseling begins. Different Ayurvedic consultants will appeal to different people. While the approaches of the Maharishi centers and of Dr. Lad are based on the same Ayurvedic principles, they have very different styles.

I found the Maharishi consultation extremely systemized, down to the computerized report I received of the doctor's

analysis. The printout was a helpful reminder of the quick interpretation I got from the doctor and health counselor at the
session. The experience struck me as another example of the
Americanization of a traditional healing art.

These centers are headed by modern medical doctors who
combine both types of medicine. They can respond with a wide
range of treatment. The Maharishi centers would be good for
people more comfortable with their Westernized and organized
approach to health. If you can afford it, you can have the support
of health counselors, regular *pancha karma* cleansing massages,
and meditation classes. You can also buy rather expensive herbal
remedies, teas, and condiments, classical elements for balancing
constitution.

My experiences with Dr. Lad, Dev Priya, and Ashwin were
very different, touching, and inspiring. Their styles would appeal
to people exposed to Eastern philosophies. In his lectures Dr.
Lad, a very spiritual and loving soul, chanted some of the original
Sanskrit phrases of Ayurveda. While I did not understand the
words, I could feel the healing wisdom and intent of the words
and his hand movements as he sang.

Dev Priya and her husband, Ashwin, on the other hand, are
working to translate the Ayurvedic metaphors into Western terms
and concepts. Their aim is to make its centuries-old wisdom,
about diet in particular, understandable to the Western point of
view. Dev Priya, an allopathic physician's assistant, has reorgan-
ized the traditional Ayurvedic approach to food using modern
nutritional criteria in their upcoming book, *Integral Nutrition*.

While consultants focus first on digestion and foods, Ayurveda also supplements nutritional programs with other therapies.
Depending on the consultant's orientation and other certifications, a client usually adds some form of massage, cleansing,
meditation, and exercise to a daily routine. Ayurveda also uses
aromatherapy, visualization, and music therapy to balance bioforces. An angry *pitta* person is told to put a dot of rose perfume
under her nose to help control emotions. *Vata* people can help
calm their nerves by listening to music.

I, as a *kapha*-dominant type, respond to the kinesthetic
treatments. I love massages. *Swedan* is an Ayurvedic cleansing
massage I tried. Sesame oil, which is considered warming and
penetrating, is rubbed into the skin to stimulate circulation. Then
an herbal steam bath sweats out the toxins. Finally, the body is

dusted with barley flour to soak up waste material, and both the flour and dead skin cells are brushed off. The treatment ends with a warm shower. I was in heaven! My sinuses cleared, my skin glowed, and I felt nurtured. Just what *kapha* types like for themselves.

Applications and Cautions

Ayurveda is a philosophy and a lifestyle as well as a medicine in India. Many aspects of it can be used to support numerous kinds of treatment programs if compatible and appropriate, as determined in consultation with your primary treatment or health care provider. Ayurveda can also be a lifestyle choice, a way to organize and enhance your daily living and health care. Once learned, its principles can be applied to every lifestyle activity. Changing lifestyle habits and diet can help with chronic complaints such as insomnia, constipation, allergies and colds, back pain, arthritis, hypertension, tension headaches, skin problems, nausea, obesity, anxiety, irritability and other emotional stresses, dyslexia, bronchitis, and digestive disorders.

Ayurveda is not recognized as a medicine in the United States. Ayurvedic practitioners are licensed instead in some other form of health care, such as chiropractic, homeopathy, acupuncture, or allopathy (modern medicine), and provide their Ayurvedic services as an adjunct to their basic services. Their Ayurvedic knowledge is offered to the client as consultation, giving guidance on managing lifestyle habits to improve general health or enhance primary treatment programs.

It is important to make sure that your practitioner is a properly licensed health care professional and that he operates within the scope of the law. This means he will have to recommend experts and services for conditions not covered in his licensed field.

Also, you must understand that Ayurveda is an entire health care system and a complete lifestyle that is foreign to many of us. While bits and pieces of Ayurvedic practices can be incorporated into your health program, a true understanding of and immersion into Ayurveda requires a great deal of motivation. You need time, energy, and a strong willingness to learn; the complexities of this system can be overwhelming. Before you begin, there are books you can read that will give you a sense of the complexity as well as the benefits and help you figure out if you are indeed ready to make the necessary commitment.

READ MORE ABOUT IT

AYURVEDA

Ayurveda: The Science of Self-Healing
by Vasant Lad
(Santa Fe: Lotus Press, 1984)

Prakruti: Your Ayurvedic Constitution
by Robert E. Svoboda
(Albuquerque, NM: Geocom, 1988)

Diet and Nutrition: A Holistic Approach
by Rudolph Ballentine, M.D.
(Honesdale, PA: the Himalayan International Institute, 1978)

Creating Health: Beyond Prevention Towards Perfection
by Deepak Chopra, M.D.
(Boston: Houghton Miffin, 1987)

Ayurvedic Medicine: The Gentle Strength of Indian Healing
by Brigit Heyn
(Wellingborough, Northamptonshire: Thorsons Publishing Group, 1987)

Health Through Balance: An Introduction to Tibetan Medicine
by Dr. Yeshi Donden
(Ithaca, NY: Snow Lion Press, 1986)

A Handbook of Ayurveda
by Vaidya Bhgwan Dash and Acarya Manfred M. Junius
(New Delhi: Concepts Publishing, 1983)

RESOURCES

The Ayurveda Institute
11311 Menaul, N.E. Suite A
Albuquerque, NM 87112
(505) 291-9793
❑ information
❑ classes
❑ counseling

Himalayan International Institute of Yoga Science and Philosophy of
the U.S.A.
RR1, Box 400
Honesdale, PA 18431
(717) 253-5551
❏ publications
❏ retreats
❏ treatments
❏ professional trainings

Maharishi Ayur-Veda Health Center
679 George Hill Road
Lancaster, MA 01523
(508) 365-4549 or 368-8660
❏ information
❏ products
❏ referral to centers

Bach Flower Remedies and Other Flower Essences

What Are Flower Remedies and Flower Essences?

Flower essence is a general term for a liquid preparation created by immersing a flower into water and exposing the preparation to sunlight or heat. This infuses the preparation with healing properties that come from the life energy and spiritual elements contained in the flower. *Flower remedy* is a term used to describe those specific products created by Dr. Edward Bach, the homeopathic physician who first developed flower preparations. He created 38 Flower Remedies in the 1930s to treat specific emotional imbalances. *Flower essences* are all the other products developed by various people since the 1960s.

Just as we consume food to nourish or use herbs to heal the physical body, flower remedies and essences are used to nourish, as well as help heal the physical body. According to developers of flower preparations, these products strengthen the individual and allow his innate spiritual powers to enhance the body's and the mind's natural healing abilities.

History and Development of Flower Remedies and Essences

Edward Bach was a bacteriologist and homeopath who turned to research when he became disillusioned with the side effects of drug therapies. Because he believed that illness is a symptom of mental or emotional imbalance, he turned away from drug treatments, retiring to the countryside in Wales to explore the healing power of nature. Reasoning that the healing effects of plants and herbs might also be captured in water drops on their flowers, he sipped the morning dew from particular flowers he found on walks through the countryside.

Bach postulated that emotions such as guilt, fear, or doubt create personality fixations, which would eventually lead to physical consequences—stress, pain, illness. He developed a remedy system using flower essences. It was based on key personality types with chronic patterns of mental or emotional imbalance that created tendencies for certain chronic diseases. Bach Flower Remedies are made of flowers found mostly in Britain.

Four decades later, an American developed essences from flowers native to northern California. Richard Katz realized that local vegetation is Nature's medicine chest and that the healing powers of flower essences were not limited to 38 English plants. He used himself as a guinea pig to prove the efficacy of each essence. A long-time student of spiritual tradition and growth psychology, Katz also created affirmations for his 72 Flower Essence Society (FES) preparations and Bach's 38 remedies.

Katz seems to have broken a conceptual dam. Flower essences have been developed and continue to be created using local flora in many locations around the globe. Like Bach, Katz made "mother stock" bottles, concentrates of single-flower essences; the practitioner would then make up remedy preparations by mixing these individual flower preparations. As the popularity of these flower essences grew in the 1980s, several more companies appeared in the marketplace with ready-to-use preparations. These premixed bottles, both single and combination flower essences, are labeled with the specific issues, attitudes, or emotional problems they are designed to affect. Each group or essence system has its own particular focus—spiritual, emotional, psychological, physical—giving individuals and practitioners a wide variety of choice. Bach Flower Remedies are the Cadillacs of the field, however. They are, in fact, currently listed as over-the-counter remedies in the *Homeopathic Pharmacopeia*.

It also must be mentioned that some of these companies market gem essences, too. These are similar liquid preparations, using the energy of precious and semiprecious stones to heal or balance energy.

How Do Flower Preparations Work?

Bach believed that the unique healing power of a plant is in its energetic property, which can reestablish the link between body and soul, nature and spirit. Disconnected, the internal disharmony and stress results in illness or self-alienation as "disease." Flower remedies, he thought, help to restore that awareness of inner connectedness or wholeness, which then energizes one's self-healing powers. Others characterize flower essences as working in much the same way, though each group has a slightly different way of describing it. Some name different levels of the self that their essences affect. For example, the Santa Fe Flower Connection women have created five groups: Emotional, Attitudinal, Spiritual, Age Group Mixtures, and General Problems. They market products such as: Changing Habits, Clearing Guilt, For Kids of Divorce, and Aura Balancing.

Most evidence and case studies on flower essences are subjective and anecdotal. People report changes in attitudes and breakthroughs in emotional issues; practitioners record observations of progress of patients who include the remedies as part of an overall treatment program.

In 1979, Michael Weisglas, Ph.D., conducted a double-blind test of Bach remedies as part of his doctoral dissertation research. Neither the subjects nor Weisglas knew beforehand who got the preparations and who got placebos. The results demonstrated that the effects observed could not be attributed to the placebo effect. In other words, the subjects in the study showed changes that could not be explained solely through the idea that getting *any* kind of treatment leads to improvement.

Those taking a four-essence combination experienced enhanced personal well-being and growth, reporting such benefits as deeper self-understanding and self-acceptance, a better sense of humor, and greater creativity. The group taking a seven-essence mix noted a decreased sense of well-being; the placebo group showed no statistically significant change. On the basis of his studies, Dr. Weisglas concluded that the effects of the essences do not depend on the beliefs or faith of the user.

How Are Flower Remedies and Essences Used?

Bach's most famous remedy is a combination of five flowers, called *Rescue Remedy*. Used in emergency situations or for trauma, Rescue Remedy helps reduce the effects of trauma and marshal the body's own healing powers. Recently, I bought some

"RR" and had it in my purse when I attended a cousin's wedding. Just before the ceremony started, a bee stung my uncle in the eyeball. I immediately administered Rescue Remedy, putting drops both in the eye and under his tongue. His eye never swelled, and the pain was minimal.

Flower remedies and essences are used by individuals as home remedies and by professionals as counseling tools. Holistic physicians, chiropractors, and other health practitioners may use the remedies as part of their practice. They are not used as a medication to cure a physical disease, but rather to gain insight, by observing a client's reaction to the administration of various essence mixtures, on the emotional or life stresses that may contribute to the origins of the illness or chronic condition.

The mixture can be determined by reading the descriptions and affirmations, by analyzing one's history and current issues or illness, by radiesthesia (use of a pendulum for psychic sensing of subtle energy radiations), or "muscle testing." In muscle testing, the client or receiver holds the bottle, or has it placed on the body. The practitioner or tester asks, silently or aloud, whether this flower is appropriate for the problem or useful for the health goal at this time. The client holds out an arm and resists while the tester gently presses on it. Muscles are tested without the bottles first. A strong or stiff muscle reaction usually (but not always) means yes, a weak one means no. In the pendulum test, a similar question is asked as the pendulum is suspended. The pattern of its swinging motion determines the answer.

Psychotherapists may choose flower essences as a creative counseling tool. "Essences can help identify and focus attention on deeply buried feelings or issues," says Lynn Rabinov Vespe, a San Francisco Bay Area psychotherapist. "It is a useful adjunct to the therapeutic process of uncovering, facing, and resolving life incidents, traumas, and decisions."

Vespe related a personal experience to illustrate:

"I was talking with a friend about a confusion in my life, [centering] around my mother. My friend, also a counselor, intuited several essences to try, and Bach's Rock Rose tested strongest. I discounted the idea at first because Rock Rose is for fear and terror." She paused to smile, thinking back to that day. "But as I thought about it, I realized I had been denying the fear of success in myself for a long time." Not wanting to see herself as afraid of anything, she had buried feelings of panic and fear so deeply that even she was not aware of them.

"I realized that testing a range of essences could be a good assessment tool, revealing feelings one might otherwise manage to ignore. Taking the essence helped me focus on and clear some deep-seated feelings."

The layperson often buys the retail bottles of flower essences for specific obstacles or issues she or he wishes to overcome. I was introduced to the Bach Remedies by a chiropractor. And I have a set of the FES essences that I sometimes share with friends when they ask for insight and support for a wide range of challenges. As essences grow in popularity, more and more seekers in the holistic and spiritual movements are making their own essences, the process or ritual of making them becoming almost as important as the end product.

Some doctors include flower remedies in a comprehensive treatment program for serious medical problems. Physicians have given cancer patients the drops to help them deal with fear of death and other strong emotions that are experienced during treatment. The remedies can also be employed to strengthen a patient's will to make vital changes in lifestyle, changes needed to help heal or prevent a disease or chronic condition. A book by Gurudas (channeled by Shirley MacLaine's psychic, Kevin Ryerson) lists in concise charts the flower essences he claims most useful to address specific diseases, organs, emotional problems, and professions.

Standard dosage is three to seven drops under the tongue, four times a day. Concentrates can be diluted in a glass of tea. Frequency, not dose, is increased to intensify the effects of treatment.

"I tell my clients to hold the drops under their tongues while opening themselves to the healing vibrations of the flowers," explains Lynn Vespe. "Then I ask them to say an affirmation, get a picture in their mind of a wanted outcome, or just think about why they are taking the essences."

Again, don't overdo the number of essences or the frequency of taking them. I have lost track of the number of flowers in home-remedy mixtures I had made up for various issues. Dealing with them simultaneously, I experienced a kind of emotional processing frenzy. While, in my experience, some essences are subtle and others faster-acting, all can eventually stimulate a sense of awareness or opportunity to address the issues to which they are particular. Be good to yourself. You don't have to confront *all* your psychological warts or life imbalances at once!

Applications and Cautions

Whether you are an individual interested in buying or making your own remedies, or the client of a practitioner who incorporates essences in her practice, there are a few important points to remember. First, flower preparations can be used one at a time or in combination. Michael Weisglas's research showed that seven or more remedies in a mixture can have negative effects—too much stimulation or too many issues stirred up at once. You should choose one or two conditions to focus on, to avoid taking on too much at once.

Whether by rational deduction, intuitive insight, or the power of the body or spirit to communicate its wishes, you should select the flower remedies or essences by testing or validating them for yourself. Each stock bottle (if using Bach or FES systems) or commercial selection should be tested individually and then in combination. If choosing by muscle testing, read the description of issues related and decide if you want to work on this aspect of yourself at this time. If a counselor chooses flowers by analyzing the client's history, matching the emotional problem with the flower's profile, or by intuition, he should also verify the mixture. Muscle testing or radiesthesia are common methods for giving voice to a client's more spiritual agreement with the choice. Incidentally, Bach Remedies' U.S. representative, Leslie Kaslof, asserts that active engagement isn't necessary for a remedy to work. He says that animals treated with Remedies get therapeutic benefits as well!

Because no toxic elements of the flowers are transferred in the preparation of a remedy or essence, you do not have to worry about possible allergic reactions. However, you should still pay attention to each flower used in the commercial combinations. They are listed on the label. Bach identified several flowers for fear, but for different kinds of fear. Some of these are grouped in one mix and may not be right for your situation. Read up on the flowers before trying a product.

READ MORE ABOUT IT

BACH FLOWER REMEDIES
AND OTHER FLOWER ESSENCES

Heal Thyself
by Edward Bach
(London: Fowler, 1931)

Bach Flower Remedies
by Philip M. Chancellor
(New Canaan, CT: Keats Publishing, 1971)

The Medical Discoveries of Edward Bach, Physician
by Nora Weeks
(New Canaan, CT: Keats Publishing, 1973)

Bach Flower Therapy: Theory and Practice
by Mechthild Scheffer
(Rochester, VT: Thorson Publishers, 1981/1987)

*Patterns of Life Force: A Review of the Life and Work of
    Dr. Edward Bach*
by Julian Barnard
(Herford, England: Bach Educational Programme, 1987)

RESOURCES

Dr. Edward Bach Healing Society
P.O. Box 320
Woodmere, NY 11598
(516) 593-2206
❏ information
❏ publications
❏ trainings
❏ products

Flower Essence Society
P.O. Box 459
Nevada City, CA 95959
(800) 548-0075 or
(916) 265-0258
❏ information
❏ classes

❏ training and certification
❏ products
❏ publications
❏ consultation
❏ research
❏ membership

Bioenergetics and Body-Oriented Psychotherapies

What Are Reichian-Based Body-Oriented Psychotherapies?

Body-oriented psychotherapy is an offshoot of traditional psychotherapy, a primary treatment for mental illness that helps individuals cope with and resolve psychological and emotional problems. The psychotherapist is a specialist in defense mechanisms—those symptoms or habits we unconsciously use to avoid feeling or realizing our internal pain and confusion. Some defense systems can include physical symptoms or psychosomatic illnesses.

There are numerous schools of personality theory and psychotherapeutic technique. The healing power of touch, used since the dawn of history, is recognized by some treatment systems and many individual therapists. Various kinds of touch—holding, massage, tapping the body—are used to reach schizophrenic and autistic children, for example. Body-oriented psychotherapies incorporate many different kinds of contact. These can range from invasive—the therapist applying strong pressure on the patient's chest—to nurturing, where the therapist gently cradles the client.

Some therapists combine classical "talk therapy" with body or movement techniques. Dance/Movement Therapy, for one, uses expressive movement exercises to uncover deeper levels of feeling or unconscious memories for therapeutic discussion. Many traditional therapists believe physical contact, however, is problematic in the therapeutic relationship. But some will recommend that clients get a massage or a Rosen Method session to increase body awareness as part of the therapeutic process.

Body-oriented psychologies treat body and mind as inseparable. They recognize that our body types and movement habits are integral parts of our personalities. A small, lithe gymnast sees and moves through life in a way a six-foot linebacker cannot. We experience ourselves (and others) differently depending on whether we are, say, chronically stiff and in pain, or flexible and vibrating with health.

Reichian theory, based on the original thinking of radical psychoanalyst Wilhelm Reich, explores the healing capabilities of the body's sexually driven "life energies." Bioenergetics is the most established and popular offshoot of the original Reichian Therapy. Hakomi Body-Oriented Psychotherapy, combining Eastern philosophy with Western body-oriented psychotherapy theories, is another example of a therapy system rooted in Reichian theory, refining Reich's original techniques into a different, more gentle orientation. Stanley Keleman's development of somatic (meaning related to the body) psychology theory illuminates "embodying" our lives, or living our experience in our whole bodies.

History and Development of Body-Oriented Psychotherapies

Turn-of-the-century European society shifted away from puritanical and Victorian repression toward a new openness.

One area in which this new freedom was manifested was a growing interest in the radical science of psychiatry. One pioneer, Dr. Georg Groddeck, proposed that sources of mental illness lay deeper than the conscious mind. In a pre-Freudian view of the unconscious, Groddeck talked about reaching the "it" (id) of a person, below his or her consciousness. He would massage, adjust, and bathe his patients, as well as prescribe exercises as part of his treatments.

Sigmund Freud changed medical and mental health history by inventing psychoanalysis, the long-term, verbal treatment of physical, psychological, and emotional problems. But while he acknowledged the body as an expression of an inner process, his theory and methods drew mental illness treatment away from massage and bone adjustment and toward dealing with unconscious dynamics.

It was his student and colleague Dr. Wilhelm Reich who developed a therapeutic perspective and methodology based on anatomy. His "vegetotherapy" (meaning a primitive, involuntary level of biological functioning) techniques emphasized freeing life energy, especially sexual energy, from chronic muscular tension.

A man ahead of his time, Reich would suffer for exposing the function of sexuality in health. In 1924, Reich became the director of Freud's first training institute for psychoanalysts. But by the late '20s he had split from his mentor and the Vienna psychoanalysts over his theoretical differences. Among other disagreements, he objected to Freud's contention that man must control his sexual drive for the good of society. Reich's radical view was that sexual instinct is the source of "life energy," which he called Orgone, and human vitality. He wanted to treat health complaints, particularly chronic conditions, by enhancing or freeing his patients' mysterious vital forces.

Reich moved from city to city in Europe, repeatedly getting into trouble for his programs and lectures on sex education and for his laboratory experiments on vital energy. America came to his rescue, when the New School for Social Research offered him an associate professorship. Reich moved to New York in 1939, establishing the Orgone Institute. He then spent the next 15 years creating devices (such as insulated boxes into which he placed people) to collect and concentrate this biological force for treatment of diseases. Reich believed restoring Orgone's natural flow in the body would help or remedy such conditions as cancer, asthma, epilepsy, and hypertension.

But Reich would run into trouble again in 1954. The federal Food and Drug Administration, alerted by a laboratory accident that exposed his assistants to radiation, and following up on complaints about his unorthodox cancer research and treatments, got an injunction to stop Reich's work. It was granted on the basis that Orgone did not exist. True to form, Reich ignored the injunction, saying the FDA did not have the scientific knowledge to judge his work. By 1956, Reich was sentenced to two years in federal prison. The FDA burned his books and papers. He died the next year of a heart attack in a Pennsylvania prison hospital.

But Reich had inspired a number of people to continue exploring his therapeutic perspective, if not his Orgone experiments. One, Stanley Keleman, writes about phenomenological (as related to human consciousness) aspects of somatic, or body-oriented, psychology. His many books explain the layers of the bodily experience, illustrating the unconscious processes that shape and give meaning to our human existence. Psychologists with practices ranging from family therapy and addiction treatment to expressive arts therapies come to Keleman's Center for Energetic Studies to gain a new perspective in their work.

Dr. Alexander Lowen rejected Orgone theory but believed in life energy, which he called "bioenergy." Lowen, along with John Pierrakos, M.D. and William Walling, M.D., established the Institute for Bioenergetic Analysis and refined Reich's basic therapeutic techniques. A prolific writer, Lowen developed Bioenergetic Analysis and Therapy and spread awareness of Reichian-based theory. Today, Bioenergetics is more widely known than Reichian Therapy. Lowen's books illustrate in depth his theoretical approach and its applications to depression, sexual functioning, general health and vitality, and other mental and physical health conditions. Pierrakos, meanwhile, left the Institute in 1974 to explore spiritual energies in healing. His Core Energetic Therapy focuses on the capacity to love and heal through an integration of body, mind, spirit, and soul.

Reichian theory continues to inspire a number of new therapeutic techniques and systems. In addition to Bioenergetics, Hakomi Therapy, developed by Ron Kurtz as a nonconfrontational refinement of Reich's practices, and Radix or Neo-Reichian Therapy are among the new therapies that acknowledge the influence of Reich's revolutionary point of view and techniques.

How Do Body-Oriented Psychotherapies Work?

Reichian and Bioenergetic Therapy spring from psychoanalytic theory. They begin with the concept of character, introduced by Freud. Character traits are consistent, habitual patterns of behavior in an individual. Shyness, aggression, and overdramatization mark defense mechanisms—different strategies, reactions, or approaches to life situations.

Reich developed character theory and added his concept of "character armoring"—chronic muscle tension resulting from unresolved emotional conflicts. He saw specific patterns of muscular tension that corresponded with particular defense mechanisms forged in early childhood. Armoring distorts or represses natural feelings, blocking three basic biological "excitations": anxiety, anger, and sexuality.

Like Freud, Reich saw sexuality as a primary force in life. But unlike Freud, Reich wanted to free that drive for pleasure and fulfillment so the individual could reach full orgasmic potential.

Lowen expanded this idea of source energy to "life of the body." He emphasized the often paradoxical relationship between mind, body, and energetic processes. Bioenergetics works with a range of repressed desires affecting adult physiology, especially loss of vibrancy in both body and life. While recognizing sexuality as important, Bioenergetics also deals with breathing, moving, feeling, and self-expression.

Reichian-based therapies aim to dissolve neurotic character structures and armoring at the deepest biological levels, restoring a free and natural energy flow in the body. Bioenergetics includes a complementary process of mobilizing the feelings expressed by the armoring. Clients reach out for what they want or need, or they hit a couch with a tennis racket to express anger or aggression. Bioenergetics also includes Reichian breathing techniques and emotional releases. "Stress postures" help fatigue-blocked muscles and joints to release pent-up emotions. A release physically tingles, the body vibrating as energy begins to flow freely. Freeing emotions can open the client to experiencing tenderness. These physical and emotional release techniques are alternated in therapy.

Reichian-based therapies employ a variety of exercises to help break through muscular-emotional armoring. Reichian and Bioenergetic techniques include:

❏ Deep breathing, letting the belly out for fuller oxygenation.

❏ Deep massaging of muscle spasm areas (armoring), while the client breathes deeply and vocalizes (yells, cries, screams).

❏ Pushing down on the chest, while the client exhales and yells.

❏ "Unmasking" or making faces, and moving parts of the face, like rolling the eyes, opening the eyes or mouth wide, and aping emotions.

❏ Exercising the gag reflex, like coughing, yawning, or opening the throat.

❏ Making bioenergetic movements, such as pounding, stamping, kicking, reaching out, shaking various limbs and body parts.

❏ Maintaining stress postures, such as leaning back over a high stool and blanket roll, with the arms out, or bending the knees and arching back until there is a release.

Hakomi Therapy has developed Reichian's rather confrontational style into a more supportive and "nourishing" set of techniques. Its operating principles are drawn from Eastern philosophy and meditation practices, such as mindfulness and nonviolence, as well as Western psychology. Creator Ron Kurtz has refined and renamed character types to highlight an individual's experience in life and strategies for coping. For example, Freud's orally fixated character becomes a dependent/endearing type,

Hakomi psychotherapists will work with a client's "state-specific memory," allowing her to consciously return to, say, an unhappy early childhood incident. The client and therapist look closely at the experience, finding solutions and options for new attitudes and behavior.

Hakomi's "Taking Over" and Stanley Keleman's "Accordion" techniques illustrate the gentler, or self-directed, new approaches to body armoring. In Taking Over, the therapist or therapy group takes over the responsibility for maintaining a chronic tension, hunching the client's shoulders around his heart, for example. The purpose is to free energy to discover and experience the feelings underneath the fear-based armoring. The Accordion technique is a process of intensifying and then slowly reducing chronic contractions. The incremental release of tension often releases long-held, literally "embodied," emotional memories.

What Happens in a Session?

A therapeutic relationship, the rapport established between client and therapist should create trust and a feeling of a safe place in which to express and explore deep emotions and fears. Therapy is a joint venture in looking at and changing the client's perspective, attitude, and behavior so her or his health improves.

Body awareness, massage, breathing, and movement techniques stimulate a new perspective on bodily shape and function. Reichian or Bioenergetic exercises work directly with breaking through body armoring that impedes the patient's functioning.

In Bioenergetics the patient uses a mat on the floor, a chair, a stool and blanket, or simply stands free. Sessions alternate between using stress position exercises to open up muscular-emotional blocks, and talking about what is happening to gain insight into those blocks.

Bioenergetics starts with a grounding and breathing exercise to focus the client. Its emphasis on "grounding"—becoming aware of one's own physical experience, rooted in the real world, identified with one's body, aware of one's sexuality, and oriented toward pleasure—distinguishes Bioenergetics from the other Reichian derivatives. Grounded people "have their feet on the ground" and know where they stand. Grounded clients can handle muscular-emotional releases, painful memory content, and psychological explorations more effectively.

To ground, a client might stand with his weight on the balls of the feet, knees slightly bent, letting go of the belly and pushing down the pelvic floor muscles with deep, audible breaths. Next, a client might slowly stretch his arms up and around, again with audible breaths.

Reich divided body armor into seven segments: eyes, mouth, neck, chest and arms, diaphragm, abdomen, and pelvis and legs. The therapist chooses exercises depending on where she perceives blocks, what issues need attention, or what seems appropriate for a particular session.

What makes this kind of psychotherapy different from bodywork releases is the specialist's skill and the depth of work in processing the content and experience of the release. Memory releases I have had on the massage table have been informative and significant. However, bringing those memories—and feelings—to a therapy session have given me a deeper and longlasting understanding of their meaning in my life.

My therapist used these tools to teach me how to cope with formerly disorienting situations. His therapeutic skills helped me build the self-confidence to use them. The therapeutic relationship supported my efforts to change my emotional and physical lifestyle—and to improve my health.

The inner emptiness I used to fill with too much or the wrong kinds of food is now filled with a new sense of myself, an awareness of how I fill that "space." When I am experiencing stress, the Accordion helps me release painful tension and sort out the feelings triggering the stress. Releasing blocks in my chest frees me to feel more open to the love and affection for and from the people in my life.

Somatic psychology has taught me about "embodiment," helping me recognize that I live in my entire body, not just in my head. My body is my friend; it give me messages about what I am experiencing. I came away from two years of body-oriented therapy sensing a new ability to move and live with more grace as long as I continue to "embody" my life.

Applications and Cautions

While severe mental illness, psychosis, and schizophrenia require more traditional treatment modalities, body-oriented psychotherapies can be appropriate for many common neuroses and problems. They can help individuals with psychoemotionally-based sexual blocks or dysfunctions, and patients with chronic physical tension, muscle spasms or pain, and psychosomatic-originated ailments.

Many individuals experience psychoemotional conflicts that are manifested in physical symptoms. These disorders can range from migraines and headaches to autoimmune conditions such as allergies. Autoimmune diseases can have a psychological aspect since symbolically, the body is turning on itself with the immune system attacking good parts as foreign germs.

Bioenergetic Analysis, especially when practiced by trained psychiatrists, is particularly successful with gastrointestinal disorders, including ulcers and spastic colon. Chronic back tension, heart disease, hypertension, and lung disorders also respond to therapy.

Body-oriented therapies not only heighten sensitivity to bodily feeling, but also release emotional energy, revitalizing the body. Releases can literally help "reshape" body structure. Chronically tight muscles that have held back repressed emotion can soften, expand, and accept more oxygen. The new vitality energizes the body's own healthy defense mechanisms and healing wisdom.

Patients undergoing verbal therapy often "get stuck." The course of treatment stalls in mind games, in blocked insight and emotions, or in other kinds of frustration. Body-awareness techniques, like dance, movement, acting, breathing, imagery, dreamwork, and hypnosis can help break through emotional barriers. The judgment of the therapist is important in determining whether, when, and what techniques may help the therapeutic process.

Reichian, bioenergetic, and the other body-oriented therapies are not for everyone. Remember that individuals form muscular armoring to protect themselves from painful memories or strong feelings. Powerful techniques designed to deepen self-awareness can awaken the individual to unaccustomed, intense feelings.

Therapists are trained to make an accurate diagnosis and devise a realistic plan of treatment. A psychotherapist's primary responsibility is to gauge the client's ego strength or ability to cope with reexperiencing feelings or pain.

Most important, therapists can create a rapport, trust, and strength in a relationship. The effects of body-oriented techniques, particularly those that work directly with defensive muscular armoring, can be unexpected and powerful. The safety and caring of a therapeutic bond can help sustain a client in those white-water rapids or floods of memories and experiences.

The experience can range from tender to momentarily terrifying, illuminating to temporarily confusing. It can be both grounding and satisfying, relieving and freeing. This is the creative edge of a good therapeutic relationship and the source of the deepest rewards of psychotherapy. Make sure you work with a qualified therapist, one who has those skills and can make those judgments.

READ MORE ABOUT IT

BIOENERGETICS AND BODY-ORIENTED PSYCHOTHERAPIES

Bioenergetics
by Alexander Lowen
(New York: Penguin Books, 1976)

The Vibrant Way to Health: A Manual of Bioenergetic Exercises
by Alexander Lowen, M.D. and Leslie Lowen
(New York: Harper & Row, 1977)

Somatic Reality
by Stanley Keleman
(Berkeley: Center Press,1979)

Selected Writings: An Introduction to Orgonomy
by Wilhelm Reich
(London: Vision, 1972)

Core Energetics: Developing the Capacity to Love and Heal
by Dr. John Pierrakos
(Mendocino, CA: Life Rhythms Publications, 1987)

Psychosomatic Medicine: Its Principles and Applications
by Franz Alexander
(New York: W.W. Norton, 1950)

Sensory Awareness
by Charles Brooks
(Great Neck, NY: Felix Morrow, 1974/1986)

RESOURCES

Institute for Bioenergetic Analysis
144 East 36th Street
New York, NY 10016
(212) 532-7742
       or
The Institute for Bioenergetics and Gestalt
1307 University Avenue
Berkeley, CA 94702
(415) 849-0101
❏ information
❏ publications
❏ workshops
❏ training and certification
❏ referrals
❏ membership
❏ research

Center for Energetic Studies
2045 Francisco Street
Berkeley, CA 94709
❏ publication
❏ workshop
❏ training

Institute of Core Energetics
115 East 23rd Street
New York, NY 10010
(212) 982-9637
       or

Core Energetics Evolution
P.O. Box 806
Mendocino, CA 95460
(707) 937-1825
❏ information
❏ publication
❏ classes
❏ training and certification
❏ research

Hakomi Institute
P.O. Box 1873
Boulder, CO 80306
(303) 443-6209
❏ information
❏ workshops
❏ publications
❏ training and certification

Graduate School for the Study of
    Human Consciousness
John F. Kennedy University
12 Altarinda Road
Orinda, CA 94563
(415) 253-2211 or 254-0105
❏ information
❏ classes and lectures
❏ accredited degrees

Biofeedback Training

What Are Biofeedback and Biofeedback Training?

Biofeedback training is a technique for learning to monitor and gain control over automatic, reflex-regulated body functions by using information obtained from various types of machines. The visual or auditory response of the machine makes physiological activities perceptible that are otherwise unconscious.

History and Development of Biofeedback

Biofeedback is an American contribution to modern holistic health care. Machines had existed earlier that were designed to show subtle physiology, including one that provided instrumental feedback on the muscles to train subjects to wiggle their ears. The real beginning of biofeedback, however, was in 1958 at the University of Chicago.

Joseph Kamiya stumbled into training students to produce alpha waves during his research on sleep and dreaming. Interested in the nature of human consciousness, he used an electroencephalograph (EEG) to detect dreaming sleep. Kamiya found that his subjects, using his feedback from the next room, were able to learn to change their states of mind and to achieve an alpha state, the most relaxed waking state.

When he moved his research to the University of California at San Francisco, he designed a machine that became the prototype for today's alpha training equipment. Subjects were hooked up to a machine they could hear. It gave a certain tone as direct feedback when the EEG indicated that they were in the alpha state. Kamiya noticed that in a few days of repeated trial and error with different frames of mind, the students learned to maintain an alpha state of "relaxed alertness" by themselves.

The concept of instrument feedback training quickly appeared in other fields with other physiological applications. Neal E. Miller at New York's Rockefeller University taught rats to regulate blood flow even though they were paralyzed with curare. Until this experiment in the late '60s, the nervous system was seen as having two distinct functions: voluntary and involuntary. Walking, speaking, and waving are all voluntary actions. Vital life maintenance functions, such as breathing, heartbeat, and blood flow were seen as entirely involuntary and automatic. Miller's and subsequent experiments proved otherwise. Elmer and Alyce Green at the Menninger Foundation in Kansas were the leaders in blood flow and hand temperature work. They showed that migraine headache sufferers were able to relieve pain by monitoring the muscle tension that caused it and learning to relax the muscles involved.

Biofeedback was used to regulate a variety of physiological functions previously thought to be uncontrollable. One of the most recent applications is for epilepsy. Maurice B. Steinman, while chief of neuropsychology research at a California hospital, discovered brain wave training could affect epileptic seizures. In 1987, I met an epileptic (at traffic school!) who had been seizure-free for seven years. She said she had controlled her epilepsy after three years of meditation, nutrition changes, and SMR (sensory-motor rhythm) biofeedback training.

Biofeedback is now a regular component of behavioral medicine and other medical applications that marry the mind and body in pursuit of health. It has ushered in a new interest in mind training and the potential to reduce reliance on drugs.

How Does Biofeedback Work?

Biofeedback is a term adapted for the medical world from the early radio industry. Feedback is an information loop set up to feed back activity results for evaluation and adjustment. A thermostat which senses the temperature of a room, then turns a furnace off or on until the desired temperature is reached, is an example of a device that uses feedback. We use it all the time. When we were children, our parents corrected and encouraged our attempts at speech until we learned to talk. We use it ourselves each time we learn to thread a needle or hit a golf ball better. Visual and auditory cues tell us what we are doing right or wrong as we observe; then we use that information on the next try.

In biofeedback training, machines monitor and mirror performance of certain bio, or bodily, functions. Heart rate; body, hand, or finger temperature; muscle tension; skin conductivity; and brain waves—all of these can be translated into auditory or visual signals via electrodes attached to the subject. Training is guided by a counselor or scientist who supports the learning process with positive encouragement and suggestions. These help the subject use the signals to modify specific activities.

The advantage of biofeedback is its promotion of self-responsibility. According to one long-time biofeedback trainer, people take the skills into daily life, learning to monitor their physiological changes. It helps them take responsibility for their own health.

The machine and the training itself do not stimulate the brain or change muscle activity. Using the machine is like stepping on the bathroom scale or looking in a mirror. It tells you how you are doing.

Subjects make the physiological changes in their own conscious or unconscious ways. Even Kamiya has a hard time explaining the exact "how," except that subjects use the constant feedback of information to change and keep changing what they do until they strike upon the right feel or action that produces results. The process is as unique and variable as the people doing it.

As for why biofeedback training helps alleviate selected medical conditions, the reasons seem to fall into two categories: physiological changes due to changes in the whole autonomic nervous system, and the positive feelings of self-control brought about by exercising personal power in a difficult or crisis situation.

Two Harvard University professors have a theory on the medical benefits of relaxation that may relate to the autonomic nervous system benefit. George S. Everly, Jr., a clinical psychologist, and Herbert Benson, M.D. (*Relaxation Response*), the director of Harvard's behavioral medicine program, think the key is in the physiological consequences of relaxation that begins in the brain.

Deep relaxation training retunes the nervous system. Specifically, it dampens the activity of certain brain chemicals (adrenergic catecholamines) which stimulate the limbic brain system. The limbic brain is evolutionarily the second layer of brain, sometimes called the emotional or mammalian brain. It produces the chemical signals that fire up our reactive, or survival, behaviors such as our "fight or flight" stress responses. It also influences, on a basic level, our need for food and sex, making us feel hunger or sexual desire—with an end to the survival of both the individual and the species.

Everly and Benson point to research that shows that the medical problems helped by relaxation training have a kind of "disorder of arousal" in this limbic circuitry. The brain is signalling a constant state of stress response and excreting limbic chemicals which may inhibit immune system functioning. The brain thinks it must gear up to fight or flee an outer battle and thus postpones or ignores its task of healing the inner sickness. Relaxing the stress response releases the body's immune forces to take on the real problem—the medical condition.

Meditation, progressive relaxation, autogenic training, imagery, and other relaxation techniques all have this benefit of shutting down the stress response and facilitating normal healings. Biofeedback training, when applied to stress reduction, focuses on very specific physiological functions with the help of a machine; it is technologically supported relaxation training.

An added benefit of direct and detailed feedback on otherwise hidden body states or functions may be the feeling of control it engenders. An emerging body of research supports the idea that enhancing one's perception of being in control of one's life has positive health effects. One study showed that giving convalescent home residents the simple power to choose their food and turn off their telephones lowered the mortality rate by 50 percent. Biofeedback training for chronic pain sufferers can empower them not only to change a body state but also to change their states of mind and, therefore, their perceptions that they are helpless, weak, and will never be "whole" again because of their pain.

Biofeedback Training Sessions

There are a wide range of both environments and equipment for trainings which can take place in hospitals, laboratories, or a counselor's or private practitioner's office. Though it is not the same as having the guidance and interpretative knowledge of a trainer, you can even use biofeedback at home with a portable version of the professional machines. The electrodes can be hooked up to your head, hands, or other parts of the body; you could be wearing a blood pressure cuff, a GSR finger ring, or a Frankensteinish headband full of wires for an EEG. It all depends on who you find to help you with your problem and what equipment they deem appropriate. However, while the instruments and applications may vary, biofeedback trainings have common elements.

For some people, it may be important from the outset to understand the connection between symptoms and the underlying physiologic mechanism targeted in the training. A tension headache, for example, can be triggered by tense muscles in the neck and shoulders. The biofeedback machine monitors these muscle groups to train the headache sufferer to recognize when this tension occurs and to ease it. Mechanical sensors take an electrical reading of the muscles, usually expressed by either sound or visual feedback—a beeping noise, say, or a bar monitor. When the muscle tenses, the beeping becomes more rapid (or the bar rises). The goal is to concentrate on what you are feeling as the reading changes, to learn to recognize both the state of tension and the state of relaxation.

It may take time to truly learn to feel the often subtle changes in muscle tension. Many people, particularly those new to healing arts exploration, are not "body aware," and haven't had much experience in concentrating on internal conditions. A good biofeedback practitioner should give you ample opportunity to repeat the training as many times as necessary to master the technique.

The trainer's role is to identify the muscles involved in the specific tension or imbalance being addressed and to act as coach, giving instructions, suggestions, and encouragement. But biofeedback is ultimately a process you control. You are the one who has to teach your muscles to relax—these are not magic machines that simply hook up and fix you. You should take time to "play" with the machine. Try tensing different muscles and see how high you can make the reading go—and at the same time notice how bad the tension makes your body feel. Experimentation helps you learn how the machine responds and how these tensions relate to your condition. It also helps to relieve the nervousness you may be feeling about being hooked up to the machine, which can impede progress.

When you first begin, your muscles may be extremely tight, and the practitioner will have to adjust the machine to a very high level of sensitivity in order to get any workable reading whatsoever. However, as the treatment sessions progress, and as your muscles have begun to ease, the machine will be adjusted to help you stretch for more subtle levels of relaxation.

Your practitioner will give you relaxation routines to practice at home. The machine will have already helped you recognize how the muscles are supposed to feel, so after initial sessions you should be able to perform the same skills without needing the beeps or bars. The idea is to wean yourself from the machine. These routines can be done both as "homework" and during tense everyday situations, helping you to translate the training from the laboratory to your daily life.

Trainings can last three weeks, three months, or three years, depending on the severity of the medical problem or the goal. Most people need a minimum of six weeks of training. Training sessions may be scheduled from once a week to daily and can last 30 to 60 minutes. Once training is over, clients schedule periodic checkups or reevaluations to monitor their progress.

Keep in mind that, like many of the healing modalities in this book, success at biofeedback can depend on three other factors:

❑ Motivation: Are you inspired enough to really work at this? Is there a hidden fear or anxiety sabotaging your motivation and ability to work with biofeedback?

❑ Expectations: Do you and your advisor have a clear idea of what your goal is or should be? Are you setting your sights too low or so high you'll be frustrated?

❑ Trainer Competence or Compatibility: There are no recipes. Each provider has a different expertise and every client a unique stress pattern. You and the trainer are like partners in a dance. Is it a fit? Do you trust and respond to your teacher and guide in this process?

Applications and Cautions

Biofeedback is used mostly for medical problems related to stress, though it is also useful for other situations like childbirth, incontinence, irregular heartbeat, and epilepsy.

Stress-related diseases include migraines and tension headaches, high blood pressure and hypertension, bruxism (teeth grinding), hyperactivity, functional colitis, Raynaud's disease, gastric and duodenal ulcers, sinus tachycardia (racing heart not related to other cardiac disease), insomnia, and muscular tics.

Other applications include relaxation training for childbirth (in Britain, mostly); neuromuscular reeducation following stroke; fecal incontinence; epilepsy; meditation; pain control; neck, back, and shoulder injuries; and severe dyshidrotic eczema (extremely itchy skin eruptions). Also, neuromuscular dysfunctioning from peripheral nerve-muscle injuries, Bell's palsy, cerebral palsy, and spinal cord injury.

There are four basic instruments used for medical applications:

❏ EMG, or Electromyograph Feedback, measures the amount of electrical charge in muscle fibers, revealing how tense they are. EMG is used for general relaxation; anxiety reduction; phobic desensitization; back, shoulder, and neck pain; tension headaches; TMJ (jaw pain); bruxism; neuromuscular reeducation (stroke patients); and cerebral palsy.

❏ Monitoring skin temperature shows vasomotor activity (ease of blood circulation controlled by constricting or relaxing the smooth muscles around the peripheral blood vessels). It is effective for migraines, Raynaud's disease, cold hands and feet, asthma, and hypertension, and is used in psychotherapy.

❏ Electrodermal or Galvanic Skin Response (GSR) is the most widely known of this class of machines, measuring subtle changes in the sympathetic nervous system which effect the moisture and therefore the conductivity of skin. It is one part of a lie detector machine, too, by the way. GSR is effective for systematic desensitization of phobias, guided imagery, stuttering, asthma, and is used in psychotherapy.

❏ The electroencephalograph, or EEG, measures brain waves to indicate the rate of rhythmic activity of your state of mind.

Beta waves mean you are awake and attentive (12–20 + hz or cycles per second) while the alpha state is relaxed and meditative (8–12 hz). Theta brain waves indicate daydreaming or twilight sleep (4–8 hz), and delta waves mean deep sleep (.5– 4 hz). The EEG is used for insomnia, obsessive-compulsive behavior, concentration and reading disorders, pain reduction, and epilepsy.

Biofeedback is not for: people taking certain kinds of medication, the old and infirm, psychotics, people with certain heart conditions, and people who can't monitor their own physiological changes. Failure to achieve results can cause more anxiety and low self-esteem than the original problem. In a few cases, the process may encourage dependency upon the trainer so that the skills are not transferred to daily life—the essential goal of biofeedback training.

READ MORE ABOUT IT

BIOFEEDBACK

Stress and the Art of Biofeedback
by Barbara B. Brown
(New York: Harper & Row, 1977)

Beyond Biofeedback
by Elmer and Alyce Green
(New York: Dell Publishing, 1977)

The Awakening Mind: Biofeedback and the Development of Higher States of Awareness
by C. Maxwell Cade and Nona Coxhead
(New York: Delacorte Press, 1979)

Biofeedback: Turning on the Power of Your Mind
by Marvin Karlins and Lewis M. Andrews
(New York: Warner Paperback Library, 1973)

The Challenge of Epilepsy
by Sally Fletcher, M.A.
(Santa Rosa, CA: Aura Publishing, 1985)

A Textbook of Biological Feedback
by Mariella Fischer-Williams
(New York: Human Sciences Press, 1986)

Resources

Association for Applied Psychophysiology and Biofeedback
10200 West 44th Avenue
Wheat Ridge, CO 80033
(303) 422-8436

❏ information (SASE)
❏ publications
❏ state association list
❏ classes
❏ membership
❏ training and certification
❏ conference

Chiropractic, Osteopathy, and Other Manipulative Therapies

What Are Chiropractic, Osteopathy, and Applied Kinesiology?

Chiropractic is the Western world's third largest primary health care profession, after medicine and dentistry. The name comes from the Greek words *cheiro* and *prakrikos,* meaning "done by hand." Chiropractors manipulate the skeletal-muscular system of the body, usually by hand. Its central modality is adjustment of the spinal column to rehabilitate normal nervous system functioning.

The scope of chiropractic practice ranges from the traditionalists, who stick mainly to spinal manipulation, to the more popular liberalists who view chiropractic as encompassing every health care tool except drugs and surgery, as limited by various state licensing laws.

The science of osteopathy, which was developed prior to the creation of chiropractic, is practiced side by side with America's orthodox medicine. Osteopaths complete a regular medical education plus an additional 500 hours of study of the muscular and skeletal systems. Like the other manipulative therapies, it focuses on keeping the body in structural balance so it can heal itself. However, osteopaths may medicate with prescription drugs as well as herbal substances and treat serious or infectious diseases.

Applied Kinesiology (A.K.) is a kind of body language that employs "muscle testing" for functional neurological evaluation. Some chiropractors use A.K. to discover and correct weak muscle patterns behind muscle spasms. A.K. features pressure point and manipulative techniques, based on Chinese medicine's acupuncture theory, and employs neurolymphatic and neurovascular reflexes as they relate to structural, chemical, and mental physiology regulating mechanisms. Created by a Michigan chiropractor, Dr. George Goodheart, Applied Kinesiology is still not completely accepted within the chiropractic field.

History and Development of Chiropractic

Manipulative massage is an ancient art, and archaeologists and historians have found proof of its regular use in daily life for over 2,000 years. A classical Greek document recorded instructions for maneuvering legs for the relief of low back problems. Hippocrates wrote about the dislocation of spinal vertebrae as the source of many diseases. Ancient American Indian hieroglyphics demonstrate "backwalking." Among the many tribes that used manipulative therapies were the Sioux and Creek in North America, and the Aztec, Mayan, and Toltec of Central America. Many Asian and Arab cultures have preserved their ancient tissue manipulation practices. Pacific island children learn to walk on the backs of adults.

In the 1700s, when Captain James Cook landed in Tahiti and complained about his rheumatic pains, the Polynesian chief sent 12 large women to his ship. Cook recounted in his ship's log that they laid him on a blanket on the floor of his cabin and proceeded to squeeze and pummel him, cracking his joints, for about 15 minutes. To Cook's surprise, he felt a little better. After four such treatments, his pain was gone.

Osteopathy was created by a Union doctor in the American Civil War who was disillusioned by medical practices of the day, such as bloodletting. Andrew Still had watched helplessly while his three children died during an outbreak of spinal meningitis. The spine, he reasoned, was the source of good health. Misaligned vertebrae, spinal lesions, or malfunctioning joints blocked blood circulation, undermining the body's ability to produce substances needed to fight disease. He remembered that he cured his childhood headaches by cracking his neck. In 1874, Still began cracking joints instead of prescribing drugs.

The founder of Chiropractic, Daniel David Palmer, had investigated the new science of Osteopathy, but developed his own point of view on the role of the spine and nerves in health. He primarily used mesmerism and magnetic healing, the precursors to hypnosis and Therapeutic Touch. However, all that changed in 1895, when Palmer gave his first manipulation treatment to a janitor.

The client, Harvey Lillard, claimed he had lost most of his hearing after straining his back at work. He had been functionally deaf for years. Palmer examined Lillard's back and found a lump along the spine, seemingly a displaced vertebra, which he forcibly manipulated back into place. Lillard reported some improvement in hearing. After several more manipulation treatments, the janitor said his hearing was back to normal.

Some investigators and detractors of chiropractic point out that all the nerves for hearing are contained within the skull. However, acupuncture theory and reports in medical literature, especially from Europe, have since alerted the West to possible connections between hypersensitivity in particular spinal regions and loss of hearing. Science is still working to pinpoint neurological evidence for such theories.

Back in the 19th century, however, Palmer cared more about developing his discovery into a treatment method than answering detractors. While he acknowledged that spinal manipulation had been around for thousands of years, he saw himself as developing the first specific levered techniques for the particular purpose of relieving spinal column and nervous system irritations. Palmer's point of view was that disease is not only due to an invasion of some entity; reduced neural signals from abnormal muscular and joint functions also reduce the body's own natural healing ability.

Palmer died in 1913, the same year that Kansas became the first state in America to license chiropractic therapists. It took more than 50 years for chiropractic to gain legal status in all 50 states and spread throughout the Western world. Of all the "alternative medicines," chiropractic seems to have had the most trouble from the orthodox medical establishment. This long-term opposition has created a large amount of resentment, misinformation, and litigation. On the other hand, the hostility of the medical establishment forced chiropractic to get its scientific act together.

Orthodox medicine's response to chiropractic's growing popularity was to create the AMA Committee on Quackery, in 1963. Documents filed in a subsequent court case revealed the committee's primary focus was to contain and eventually to eliminate chiropractic as a medical practice. Labeling chiropractic as "an unscientific cult," the American Medical Association barred its members from associating with or referring clients to a chiropractic doctor.

But the chiropractic profession still managed to thrive. In

1974, Congress voted to allow chiropractic treatment to be covered by Medicare. The U.S. Commission on Education also formally recognized the American Chiropractic Association as the accrediting agency for chiropractic education. Chiropractic students and institutions were then able to receive federal funding.

Chiropractors began filing state and federal lawsuits alleging that the AMA, the American Hospital Association (AHA), and various other medical associations had violated antitrust laws to monopolize American health care. The AMA responded by allowing its members to associate with any legally sanctioned health care professional, including chiropractors, and by officially ceasing to call chiropractic "unscientific." In 1987, the AHA allowed member hospitals to grant licensed chiropractors access to hospital facilities for a limited range of services.

In the meantime, chiropractic associations and colleges have stepped up scientific and medical research to meet orthodox medicine on its own ground. Palmer College of Chiropractic-West in San Jose, California, sponsors research conferences and publishes 60 scientific papers annually.

While realistic enough to know that chiropractic cannot match orthodox medicine's crisis intervention techniques, chiropractors are determined to carve out and maintain their niche in the health care field. As 30 percent of worker's compensation claims involve back injuries, chiropractic is proving itself cost-effective. As an example, a 1988 study looked at 20,000 cases in Florida. Injured employees receiving chiropractic therapy returned to work three times faster than those receiving medical treatment. Total cost savings for chiropractic, compared to medical care, were estimated at up to 50 percent.

In the meantime, Applied Kinesiology, developed in the 1960s by chiropractor George Goodheart, has broken out of the chiropractic field and inspired two do-it-yourself systems. One of Goodheart's students and colleagues, John F. Thie, created a simplified muscle testing treatment system for the layperson to use as preventive medicine. Thie sees his *Touch for Health* as an opportunity for families to share a new kind of "touching"—one that is healing rather than punitive or sexual.

John Diamond, M.D. has created Behavioral Kinesiology (B.K.) to help individuals cope with environmental and lifestyle factors that affect stamina. He combined basic A.K. testing techniques with his knowledge of psychiatry, psychosomatic medicine, kinesiology, preventive medicine, and the humanities. B.K., or Life Energy techniques, focuses on the role that the thymus, a gland system in the upper chest and neck, plays in overall health and body immunity.

How Does Chiropractic Work?

Manipulative therapies intervene when the body can't marshal its own ability to return to a healthy equilibrium, or homeostasis. Chiropractic is best used for pain and disorders before the body has deteriorated into a pathological or disease state. The conservative view in chiropractic theory believes that when functional problems develop into a pathological condition, patients usually need the swift and specific intervention of orthodox medicine. More liberal practitioners, however, will work on some acute conditions just after onset, looking beyond the symptoms to possible root causes present before the "dis-ease" deteriorated into disease.

Chiropractic looks for *subluxations* (partially misaligned and biochemically dysfunctional vertebrae) and other joints off-center that may be impinging upon normal neurological functioning. M.S.I. Dhami, associate professor of toxicology at Palmer College of Chiropractic-West, points out that chiropractic may influence neurohormonal control of the body. That is, malfunctioning nerve impulses may reduce electrochemical signals regulating beta-endorphins and other endogenous analgesics (natural painkillers produced in the brain).

Pain is the body's signal of distress or dysfunction. Caught early enough, it can be treated with chiropractic adjustment that may help put the body's own healing mechanisms back on track. When the pain is ignored, the neurohormonal immune system can't produce its own chemicals in appropriate amounts to solve the problem, and the body begins to spiral down into a disease state.

Chiropractic does not discount germ theory but instead stresses the concept of "susceptible host," an individual's predisposition to disease. Heredity, environmental pathogens (bacteria and other disease-causing substances), nutritional habits, subluxations, life stress factors, and learned responses to stress—all contribute to case assessment.

Chiropractors look for muscular and skeletal trauma from falls and accidents, strains and sprains. They note postural and occupational distortion that may induce abnormal joint function or muscle *tonus* (partial contraction). They ask about physical and mental stress. Pain can signal neurological disturbances, vascular congestion, mechanical malfunctions, and physical or psychological ailments.

William Meeker, Associate Dean of Research at Palmer West, says chiropractic treatment probably works on three levels:

❏ Mechanical/Anatomical: restoring movement by improving anatomical relationships and functions through a variety of spinal manipulation and joint mobilization techniques.

❏ Neurological/Reflexive: specific soft and hard tissue (joint muscles and fascia) manipulations that change nerve signaling patterns and, therefore, physiological functioning.

❏ Mental/Emotional Role: the healing aspects of human contact, its hands-on methodology, and its effects on the mind and motivation of a patient.

A.K.'s neuroreflective techniques address somatic-visceral complaints, such as an ileocecal valve spasm, abnormal contractions of the muscular gateway between the small and large intestines. Stuck open, the valve can let food material from the colon leak back into the small intestine, literally poisoning the patient. A chiropractor may stop the spasm by holding three points on the inside of the right leg and ankle to relieve nausea, headache, or abdominal pain.

What Happens at a Chiropractic Session?

Chiropractic has two philosophical and professional camps. The more traditional practitioners, called "straights" or conservatives, limit their therapy to adjusting the spine. The more liberal, called "mixers"or liberals, add complementary or auxiliary treatments, such as nutritional supplements, relaxation techniques, and diet counseling.

Chiropractic continues to develop as a scientific health care system, employing any one of more than 100 manipulative techniques. Twelve or so basic manipulations are taught at the various training schools. These range from the standard Sacra-Occipital Technique (SOT) and popular diversified methods of joint adjustments, to the gentle Thompson or trigger point techniques. Diagnostic techniques involve use of A.K., thermography (using a heat-sensing wheel), and X rays.

A visit to a chiropractor may involve full body X rays and a few bones manually pushed back into place, or may include diagnosis and treatment by the soft tissue manipulations of Applied Kinesiology. Or you may begin a program drawing from a variety of techniques that include remedial exercises to strengthen weak muscles or correct posture, physiotherapy, hydrotherapy, heat treatments, braces, yoga, massage, or acupressure. Some chiropractors may recommend or use biofeedback or other relaxation techniques, breathing exercises, vitamins and other supplements, or special diets focusing on allergies or Ayurvedic nutrition.

I have experienced the two extremes of chiropractic technique. A horseback riding accident compressed my spine and sent me to my first chiropractor. During a long course of treatment, which began with three adjustments a week for several weeks, this chiropractor switched from a hands-on methodology to machines. He ran a heat-sensing wheel down my spine for a scientific indication of abnormal temperature. Heat indicates inflammation and reduced nerve impulses from pinched nerves due to subluxed or misaligned vertebrae.

He then began making my spinal adjustments with what I called his "thumper," a hand-held mechanical device that adjusts by using shock or impact. It hurt. So do many hands-on adjustments, but each "shot" hurt my ears, too. Plus he had insisted on initial full body X rays and now planned a follow-up series, despite my concerns about radiation.

Finally, I found his practice/office management system, which included getting patients to sign contracts for treatment, off-putting. I realized I preferred a fluid, healing patient-doctor relationship with a person, not machines. I looked for another doctor.

Fortunately, I had experienced the benefits of adjustment in his early treatments before being turned off by that chiropractor's withdrawal behind machines. I was convinced of chiropractic's usefulness in my overall health care program. After trying several other practitioners, I found a chiropractor who I knew could be one of my primary care providers. Several years later, he still is.

I settled on Dr. Mitchell Corwin because he uses muscle-testing diagnostics instead of X rays. I had progressed to the other end of the chiropractic spectrum, from machines to Applied Kinesiology. Trained in "Touch for Health" myself, I knew that in the right hands muscle testing could be an effective dialogue between the body and therapist.

What makes Mitchell a typically good practitioner is his mixture of scientist and artist, technician and intuitionist. He doesn't just fix me up after roller skating accidents or stressed-out days at work. He teaches me about myself and how my body works.

For instance, he pointed out that I experience a major stress reaction, called the Dural Defense Posture of the spine. When I came in tense, terse, headachy, and fatigued, he showed me how I had literally tucked my tailbone between my legs and clamped down the muscles of my face, around my cranium, and in my jaw. I can now feel when I have had this reaction, and I've learned a few ways to relieve it, or to know when to come in for an adjustment rather than trying to let it slowly unwind.

He has been pursuing scientific, clinical study of the controversial system, Neural Organization Technique (N.O.T.), which addresses neurological dysfunction such as dyslexia and other learning disabilities, autism, and Down's syndrome. I like being an unofficial guinea pig (my words, not his). He included me in his learning process, said my feedback was interesting, and helped me feel less stressed when I was reading and speaking. We both learned, which I found very rewarding.

Most important, he stopped to listen. His willingness to answer my many questions, patience in explaining what he was doing, tact in correcting misconceptions about his work or my condition, and openness to my feedback engendered trust. This client-doctor relationship energized my faith in my ability to heal and take care of myself.

Applications and Cautions

Chiropractic is primarily used as therapy for mechanical dysfunctions, such as traumatized muscles and joints. It is very popular with people who experience low back pain, slipped disks, and sports injuries. Clients are treated for bad posture, sprained muscles and ligaments, and accident-related injuries. Chiropractic has also helped rheumatic and arthritic conditions of neuromuscular or vascular origin affecting both the spine and limbs.

Chiropractors treat neuritis, lumbago, sciatica, neuralgia, and knee, hip, and muscular pains. Some chiropractors also excel in treating dysfunctions with psychosomatic origins, such as migraines and other headaches, neurosis, conditions due to stress, and some asthma conditions. They also can address visceral dysfunctions affected by irritation of the autonomic nervous system.

Chiropractic is not good for all pain and discomfort. Initial examination must determine that the pain, such as low back pain, is due to a functional disorder and not a disease of the internal organs. While orthodox medicine questions chiropractic's diagnostic accuracy or skills, competent chiropractic doctors will refer a client to a medical practitioner for further diagnostic studies if there is a possibility that the condition is pathologic.

Some chiropractors use full body X rays. There is a trade-off for this diagnostic security. Low dosage or not, it is radiation.

Finally, remember that chiropractic treatment involves pushing, pulling, and leveraging muscle against bone against muscle. In the hands of a less than skilled practitioner, clients can sustain minor strains and sprains—or worse. While a Consumers Union survey found only 12 cases of severe strokes induced by chiropractic adjustment between 1947 and 1976, it qualified this statistic with the opinion that incidents of injury may be underreported in the industry. Potential severe complications also include fractures, spinal disk rupture, and paraplegia, it says. Once again, it is crucial that you take great care in choosing a certified, experienced practitioner whose clients will confirm his or her skill and effectiveness.

READ MORE ABOUT IT

CHIROPRACTIC AND OTHER MANIPULATIVE THERAPIES

Chiropractic Speaks Out: A Reply to Medical Propaganda, Bigotry, and Ignorance.
by Chester A. Wilks, D.C.
(Park Ridge, IL: Wilks Publishing, 1973)

Your Body Doesn't Lie
by John Diamond, M.D.
(New York: Warner Books, 1979)

Life Energy
by John Diamond, M.D.
(New York: Dodd, Mead, 1985)

Health Quackery: Consumer Union's Report on False Health Claims,
Worthless Remedies, and Unproven Therapies.
Edited by Consumer Reports Books Editors
(Mount Vernon, NY: Consumers Union, 1980)

Touch for Health: A New Approach to Restoring Our Natural Energies
by John F. Thie, D.C.
(Marina del Rey, CA: Devorss, 1973/1979)

Alternatives in Healing
by Simon and Steven J. Finando
(New York: New American Library, 1989)

RESOURCES

American Chiropractic Association
1701 Clarendon Blvd.
Arlington, VA 22209
(703) 276-8800
❑ information
❑ practitioners
❑ publications
❑ research and professional training

International Chiropractic Association
1110 North Glebe Road, Suite 1000
Arlington, VA 22201
(800) 423-4690
(703) 528-5000
❑ information
❑ publications

American Osteopathy Association
142 East Ontario
Chicago, IL 60611
(800) 621-1773 or (312) 280-5800

❏ information
❏ state association list
❏ publications
❏ certification

International College of Applied Kinesiology, U.S.A.
P.O. Box 25276
Shawnee Mission, KS 66225
(913) 648-2828
❏ information
❏ referrals
❏ publications
❏ classes and certification
❏ membership

Touch for Health Foundation
1174 North Lake Avenue
Pasadena, CA 91104-3797
(818) 794-1181
❏ information
❏ trainings and certification
❏ publications and products

Colonics
or Colon
Hydrotherapy

What Is a Colonic?

Colonics is the irrigation of the large intestine with water under gentle pressure to wash out or detoxify it of stagnated fecal material; it is a full intestinal enema. Regular enemas usually only wash the last part of the colon—the rectum and the descending colon. In a colonic, the water is infused via a tube inserted at the anus, and the dislodged waste material leaves via the same tube. Colonics is also called colon hydrotherapy, colon irrigation, and colon lavage.

History and Development of Colon Irrigation

The literature is pretty sketchy on the history and development of colonics. It is not a subject discussed in public with comfort. Recently, however, legal controversy and the AIDS crisis has put modern proponents of colonics on the alert. Practitioners are making more effort to inform people of the benefits of colonics, as well as to reduce the risk of injury and infection.

It seems the Egyptians were the first to describe the infusion of aqueous substances into the intestine through the anus. The *Ebers Papyrus,* a 1500 B.C. document, includes this treatment in its description of medical practices of the time. The colonics literature also points out that Hippocrates, the father of modern medicine, mentioned enemas as therapy for fever. In the second century A.D., Galen, another foundational figure in medicine, referred to the use of enemas, too.

The Essences, an early Christian aesthetic community, used water therapy to rid the body of uncleanliness and diseases that defile the body as the temple of the soul.

Colonics has been one of the healing techniques used by chiropractors and naturopaths during this century. In California, chiropractors are lobbying against an interpretation of medical practice laws that would limit the practice of colon hydrotherapy to licensed physicians.

Today, the colon hydrotherapy industry uses purified water and has developed disposable colonic equipment parts. Throwaway tubes ensure clients of more safety than even normal sterilization practices in this age of communicable diseases.

How Does Colon Hydrotherapy Work?

The colon—part of the large intestine and a key part of the digestive system—is the body's major eliminative organ. It is the last place where water and nutrients from the food we eat can be digested and absorbed by the body. Bacteria in the colon performs this process. From the colon, waste material moves on to the rectum and anus, where it is discharged. One major purpose of the colon is to draw moisture out of the stool. It hydrates the body, contributing water and electrolytes (biochemical ions necessary for all nerve-cell transmission to blood plasma via the lymph system). But as a last resort, the body will draw out the moisture even if it is from feces overrun with bacteria.

The drier the feces, the harder they are to move along, and the more likely they are to enhance bacterial growth. These are not the "friendly" kind of bacteria that aid in the digestion and absorption of nutrients to nourish the body. Rather, they create toxins and gas which, absorbed by the body, can poison it. It is the difference between absorbing pure saline or toxic waste water into your system. In the extreme, it can cause toxemia. The absorption of any amount of toxins can affect the immune system and contribute to ill health.

If the colon is weak or dysfunctioning—and does not properly send waste onto the rectum—the body builds up an overload of waste material. Then the other elimination organs—the liver, kidney, skin, and lungs—must work even harder to eliminate waste from the body. There are several general causes for waste buildup:

❑ Bad dietary habits: eating low fiber, high fat foods; eating too much or too quicky; poor food combinations (eating foods that need competing digestive enzymes, like the classic American meat-and-potatoes dinner, so some of it sits and begins to decompose); drinking large quantities of liquids at meals that dilute digestive enzymes.

☐ Not enough water: drinking coffee, tea, alcohol or colas that contain caffeine that dehydrates the stool.

☐ Emotional stress: the "fight or flight" stress reaction to anger, frustration, fear, overwork, and unhappy life circumstances all involve the release of adrenaline. Adrenaline triggers defensive needs, like an alert mind and tense muscles, but slows or shuts down "non-essential systems" like digestion and elimination.

☐ Psychological prohibitions: negative feelings, ideas, or memories about elimination left over from the toilet training years.

☐ Bad habits as adults: ignoring the call of nature or being in jobs that don't allow you to go to the bathroom when you feel the need. This ruins the tone of the segmoid and rectum muscles—the parts that push out the feces.

☐ Illness: long bed rest, anesthetic for an operation, or pain medication can result in sluggish body functions.

☐ Physical stress or defects: genetic or accidental impairment of nerve functioning or spinal misalignment.

Whatever the cause, a colonic removes the stagnated fecal material. The therapist controls the flow of water into the large intestine so the pressure does not exceed ¼ to 1½ p.s.i. (pounds per square inch). The water dislodges, dilutes, and removes feces and bacteria that have built up in the colon. The pressure of the water itself stimulates the intestines to dislodge impacted pieces of hard, dry feces stuck in the twisted intestinal wall. The use of cool and warm water causes the intestinal walls to relax and contract the involuntary muscles. This wavelike rhythm of contraction-relaxation is called peristalsis, and it is this that normally moves the contents of the colon through to the rectum and anus. During this irrigation, massaging the abdomen also helps move the constipated material. A colonic can exercise the large intestines, toning the wall of the colon and promoting peristalsis, making your bowel movements both easy and regular.

In a colonic, the outflow of water takes with it feces, gas, mucus, and the bacteria that grow on the decomposing feces.

The cleaner the inside of the colon, the more surface area there is to absorb water and electrolytes. Healthy peristalsis and regular bowel movements enhance the length of time it takes the food to go through the entire intestine, allowing more nutrients to be absorbed and keeping feces from decaying.

What Happens in a Session

While colonics is one of the healing arts I use often while facing a health challenge, it was the hardest first session I can remember. All my feelings about modesty, privacy, and being invaded came up just thinking about finding a colon hydrotherapist. I interviewed several people before choosing one for my initial session.

Usually, you lie on your back on a table with your knees bent. My colonic hydrotherapist had me wear an old pair of men's pajama bottoms. Other therapists use sheets to cover the client for modesty's sake. The important thing is that she made me feel comfortable and at ease.

The tube is gently inserted in the anus and water is slowly infused into the intestine. You may or may not feel the pressure or the temperature of the water at first. It depends on how sensitive you are or how aware you want to be. It is important to pay attention, however, since you need to give the therapist feedback on whether the water is too warm or cool or the pressure uncomfortable. Sometimes in first sessions, it takes a bit of time before the large intestine starts to release. Occasionally, the rectum needs to be cleared before the intestine can be filled. It may be so stagnated that peristalsis is not so easily stimulated or you might be so nervous that natural peristalsis shuts down. Relax.

Sessions are usually 45 to 50 minutes. Most therapists will schedule an hour or more for the first session in case it takes a little longer for the intestines to begin to release. Some colonic therapists will put a heating pad on the abdomen or small of the back or massage the abdomen to help stimulate the colon to release. Breathing, imagery, and meditation can also help.

I have never experienced real pain and only mild discomfort during intense releases. My early colonics cleared out *years* of encrusted feces and some pockets of very warm, infected or decomposed material. Those releases felt like a few minutes of turista—an urgent feeling of having to go. One practitioner told me that the older the feces (the longer they have been in the colon) the warmer they feel.

Another thing about having a colonic: "It's like turning over ripe compost—it smells!" says Nancy Gardner, president of the California Colon Hygienist Society and a former surgical nurse who has been doing colonics for over a decade. I have had some pretty hot stuff come out. It made me very aware of the effects of poor diet and a high-stress work life. I felt very light, a kind of internal calm or quietness after those kinds of releases. I know I lost three or four pounds from the clearing of my intestines in the first three sessions.

Once, at the end of a series of colonics, I came to the session needing to talk about a problem. I was very upset about an incident in a current relationship that reminded me of a similar trauma in my young adulthood. As I talked about it, I experienced a tremendous release of impacted material. It was like having a bout of diarrhea. It felt like a sudden release of energy that had literally been captured in my intestines all that time. I shook as the energy was released and cried the tears I had not allowed myself to show back then. It is possible to have a release like this with an emotional or energetic component during a colonic: it is a kind of cleansing crisis.

Applications and Cautions

A cleansing crisis is like a healing crisis, you may seem to get a little worse before getting better. One of the important cautions about colonics is that cleaning out the colon can stimulate a general cleansing in the body. With the intestines clearer and able to process more material, with the colon walls cleaner and able to absorb more water and electrolytes that enhance the immune system, the body may decide to clean house. A clean colon lightens the burden on other organ systems that eliminate waste and poisons.

Diarrhea, intestinal or stomach flu, and even vomiting can be signs that these other organs are throwing off extra waste matter from your system. It is important to find a primary care provider who understands the holistic approach to the body and health, who can evaluate what is happening to you. Work with your doctor or care provider to determine if and when to apply colonics, and how often. And, should such symptoms arise, he or she can help determine the cause.

Gardner also warns us of another possible side effect of colonics. "A colonic can wipe out the friendly bacteria or electrolytes from the large intestines during the time of the colonic. It is important to replace them by drinking plenty of water and taking supplements such as potassium, cell salts, or acidophilus," she explains.

The California Colon Hygienist Society and other colonics professionals recommend a series of questions to ask to help you evaluate a potential colon therapist:

❑ Ask about training and certification. There are several organizations, state by state, that certify Colonic Therapists. These agencies test individual practitioners on anatomy and physiology, diseases related to the colon, contra-indications for colonics, safety and sanitation procedures, and ethics.

❑ Choose someone who works under the supervision of a primary care provider or doctor who is certified, trained, or at least educated in colon hygiene. Some chiropractic schools include colonics in their curriculum. Ask the supervisor what are the benefits and potential side effects of colon hydrotherapy.

❑ Check the water used, its source, and how it is purified. Tap water in some areas is not fit to drink and thus not fit for your intestines to drink either. Chlorinated water may kill off the good bacteria in the colon. Ask what kind of purification system is used, how often the filter is changed, and what it filters out. Check that the system filters out heavy metals (from rusty pipes, especially) and bacteria, such as Giardia.

❑ Ask if disposable parts are available, to prevent the risk of infection from a previous client. It may cost you more per treatment ($3–5) but is worth it.

Once you are assured of safe treatment, colonics has several applications you may consider:

❑ Intestinal dysfunction: for relief of constipation, diarrhea, diverticulitis, and parasitic infestation.

❏ Chronic diseases: conditions such as candida that, directly or indirectly, may involve bacterial poisons absorbed by the colon or the colon's ability to eliminate waste.

❏ General toning of the intestinal muscles and elimination system may have beneficial effects on other body systems, especially lymph and blood circulation, skin, eyes, muscles and joints, and the genitourinary tract.

❏ Major diseases of other eliminative organs: improving the colon's performance relieves the burden on them. For example, cleansing the colon may reduce stress on the liver or gallbladder, if already weakened from disease, by eliminating toxins these organs would otherwise have to neutralize.

❏ Slow transit time: returning to normal the time it takes for food to be broken down, absorbed, and eliminated means bacteria won't have the opportunity to grow on the decaying feces.

❏ Enhancing the cleansing effect of fasting: first, to clear the intestines *before* starting a fast so toxins released during the fast can be eliminated rather than circulated back into the bloodstream. Second, because the intestine is empty (you are ingesting only liquids) a colonic *during* fasting gives it even more of a wash.

❏ Nutrient enema or colonic: adding aloe vera, wheatgrass, or oxygen to the water helps heal the intestinal wall. Those nutrients feed the body through the intestine. As with the water, purity here is essential and you're certainly allowed to voice your concerns about this to the therapist. Check this idea out with your primary care provider. Caution: too much oxygen can cause a headache.

Most colonic therapists will also make recommendations for a more complete cleansing program. Besides fasting, they may suggest saunas to sweat out impurities through the skin; hot tub soaks and dry brush massages; deep breathing or exercise to increase oxygen to the body and blood; drinking lots of clean water to flush out the kidneys and lubricate the elimination system; and a liver-gallbladder flush of some sort to give those organs a chance to release their loads (see Polarity). Some practitioners may suggest adding intestinal brushing products to the colonic, such as psyllium seeds. Stress reduction tech-niques—yoga, meditation, or aerobic exercise—might also be suggested. They may recommend dietary changes such as eating more grains and fibers, less fat and dairy, less red meat or no meat altogether, and using food combinations to enhance nutrient absorption. And they might suggest curbing mucus-forming foods, such as bread and ice cream, and cutting out any foods to which you are allergic.

Any and all of the suggestions they make are yours to follow or not. It is important to check with your doctor or primary care provider before incorporating colonics or other changes into your health routine.

READ MORE ABOUT IT

COLONICS OR COLON HYDROTHERAPY

Healing Within: The Complete Colon Health Guide
by Stanley Weinberger
(Larkspur, CA: Colon Health Center, 1988)

Colon Health: The Key to Vibrant Life
by Norman W. Walker, D.Sc., Ph.D.
(Phoenix: O'Sullivan Woodside, 1979)

RESOURCES

California Colonic Hygienist Society
Mill Valley, CA
(415) 383-7224

The Feldenkrais Method

What Are Functional Integration and Awareness Through Movement?

The Feldenkrais Method is a new kind of learning system that uses movement as a model and means to facilitate creating a new sense of one's self as a physical being. Feldenkrais is taught in private sessions, called Functional Integration, or in group sessions, called Awareness Through Movement. Both focus on developing ease of movement in every part of the body. They teach pupils to notice how they are using, or misusing, their bodies. From this awareness comes the ability to change and develop more healthful ways of using the body. The method's aim is to restore the ability to move as freely and spontaneously as a child, liberated from bad body habits that contribute to a myriad of health problems.

History and Development of the Feldenkrais Method

Moshe Feldenkrais was a Russian-born Israeli physicist and engineer. He left Palestine to earn his doctorate at the Sorbonne in Paris and was working on an atomic development project when Hitler invaded France. Escaping across the channel to England in 1940, he spent the rest of the war working for the British Admiralty on antisubmarine technology.

It was during this period in Britain that Feldenkrais began to develop his method. A black belt who founded the first judo school in Europe, Feldenkrais had also been an avid soccer player. In England, an old knee injury kept flaring up. Doctors recommended surgery that only had a 50 percent chance of success. Frustrated, Feldenkrais decided instead to teach himself how to walk without pain.

138

This set him on his lifelong study of the mechanics of the body and its relation to learning and behavior. After the war, he studied anatomy, physiology, psychology, and anthropology. He learned about neurology and the relationship between movement and human development. He also worked with F. M. Alexander (the Alexander Technique) and explored Gurdjieff's spiritual philosophy, Freud's psychology, and yoga.

In 1947, Feldenkrais laid out the foundations of his bodywork system in *Body and Mature Behavior: A Study of Anxiety, Sex, Gravitation and Learning*. Shortly thereafter, he returned to Israel to direct its Electronic Department of Defense. He also began formalizing "Functional Integration" and "Awareness Through Movement" as the two components of his Method.

Over the next 35 years, Feldenkrais taught thousands of pupils all over the world and conducted several trainings for teachers, including two in the United States. Since his death in 1985, Feldenkrais teachers have organized themselves into guilds in the U.S., France, Germany, and Australia. The American-based guild has taken leadership in directing training programs for new teachers.

The work continues to develop and explore some interesting directions. For instance, one of Feldenkrais's first U.S.-certified teachers, Frank Wildman, traveled to Australia in the early '80s to teach psychologists this new perspective on learning. They did not accept the program as readily as Wildman had hoped. However, one participant invited him to present his findings to senior physical therapists in Sydney. Those allied medical workers, who deal with the aftermath of trauma and neurological disease, did respond quite positively. Wildman now spends four to six months of the year in Australia training them at a top physiotherapy school. His approach to the Feldenkrais Method as a neurologically-based system for education—not bodywork—has gained it growing acceptance in the Australian medical world.

How Does the Feldenkrais Method Work?

The key to the Feldenkrais Method is awareness—of the skeleton and its muscles, and of its orientation and movement in space. Feldenkrais saw humans as having four states of being: asleep, awake, conscious, and aware. Consciousness is a higher aspect of wakefulness. Awareness is the combination of consciousness with knowledge.

Feldenkrais believed that awareness, an attentiveness to both one's internal experience and external environment, is developed through experience. So he set about creating learning situations with his simple movement exercises to give his students that experience. Movement is the other key to his method.

To Feldenkrais, movement is the essence of life. Every thought and emotion finds expression in various movements. From the firing of synapses in the brain and the narrowing of our pupils at an idea, to a smile or doubling over with laughter at a joke, there are many kinds of movements that express our feelings and attitudes.

Sometimes these movements are the result of some imbalance and cause us pain. For example, years of hunched shoulders in response to parental bickering not only distort the body but also depress emotions and self-image. Feldenkrais teachers would look at a person with hunched shoulders and see an emotional asymmetry imprinted on the brain.

Each repeated movement sends a signal, recording an image of that movement on the brain. Restricted movements fix distorted images in the mind. The messages are stored and later released, duplicating those kinds of restricted movements, rather than the free and natural actions that are our potential. The brain, through the repeated action of pulling up the shoulders, has learned to return signals to the body to hold that shape.

Awareness of our movements can help us modify the brain's signals. Debilitations of aging and twisted bones or a curved spine are not necessarily fixed and inevitable. Wildman says that "the degree to which a body can learn is the degree to which a body can change."

Feldenkrais works to give the brain, and therefore the body, new messages, new images and patterns for movement. Relearning simple and then increasingly more complex movements can rewrite the programming in the mental computer. The task is to help clients free themselves from old patterns of distorted position and movement and learn to transmit new patterns and ways of moving to their bodies. The goal is to regain the potential to move with grace and freedom, like babies exploring their world, effortlessly.

Some clients turn to the Feldenkrais Method to work on

distorted movement patterns they developed as adults, while others use it to unravel and relearn habits imprinted from infancy. Some challenges are neurological, some orthopedic, and some psychological. All are met with the understanding that the task is to discover the body's learning potential, whatever that may be.

Another important feature of the Feldenkrais Method is that clients take responsibility for themselves. Clients do the exercises to understand how they operate their bodies and then learn to live effortlessly in accordance to their own natural constitutions and abilities. Octogenerians will probably not be able to bench press 300 pounds, but seniors can learn to move with much greater ease and energy.

Wildman tells a story about a young woman who wanted to take an Awareness Through Movement class but could only attend at a senior group time. Huffing and puffing after the first 15 minutes of standing and sitting, she was flabbergasted to see that the 70- and 80-year-olds who had been attending the class for several semesters could do the exercises with ease.

Wildman calls this moving "smarter." "Rather than expend *more* effort to do what we used to do, we can become more efficient in how we use our bodies," he explains. "Instead of building muscle mass to *force* the body to perform, one can reorganize how he or she moves. Cleverness, not force, is the idea.

"We are using more of the brain's capacity and learning to be more sensitive to what we are doing with our bodies. With Feldenkrais, you feel and learn. We as teachers create conditions—teach exercises or movement tasks—so you, the pupil, can become aware of what you are doing." Clients learn not just to stretch but also to release muscles *and* reorganize how to move body parts.

What Happens in a Session?

Whether you enroll in Awareness Through Movement, the group work, or take a series of individually tailored sessions, Functional Integration, you learn on the floor. Exercises are performed in a prone or supine position to reduce the effects of gravity on joints and the feet. Since we do most of our waking activities upright, lying down to think and move allows our brains to help break down some of our patterned muscular responses. It also allows us to feel our movements differently, and *that* is the idea.

Lessons start with very simple movements, such as extending and flexing the foot. My first exercise was to lie on my back with knees bent so my feet were close to my body and then *slowly* lower my knees to one side and then the other. We were gently reminded to keep our attention on our internal experiences, to sense just what our legs and muscles are doing. The teacher directed us to notice other parts and the whole of our bodies. What parts were participating in this movement task? Were they necessary to the movement? I discovered that I use my shoulders and upper arms in movements that have nothing to do with them.

The lessons build on simple, everyday actions and specific tasks. Sitting is a habitual movement, one that we rarely think about as we do it. Feldenkrais pupils practice sitting and standing over and over again, noticing the efforts they make to get up. Do they stiffen their necks and lead with their chins? What parts of the body also tense when they just think about getting up?

I learned that I would try to force myself up from the ground by pressing my legs down too early, before balancing myself over my feet. This seems to be a common way people have mislearned the simple movement of getting up from a chair. In class, I learned to rock forward, pushing straight up with just the lower part of my legs. Then I did not have to use my back, chest, and neck to drag myself to a stand. When I understood how to simplify and free my movements, I was able to conserve energy and avoid strain.

The specific little lessons were helpful, but not as rewarding as my achieving a new awareness that I could reorganize myself. I became more sensitive, more observant of my movements. And I could "sense out" how to perform some of them differently. However, the guidance and reflection of the teacher is invaluable. If you want to work with serious orthopedic, neurological, or psychologically-based movement challenges, the private lessons would be most helpful.

Applications and Cautions

Feldenkrais is so accessible and adaptable, so simple and self-directed, that almost anyone can do it. The supple yoga devotee, the developed athlete, the physically disadvantaged, and the elderly—all can find some level of benefit, because it is not simply a physical training. It is a training of the mind, as well.

Moshe Feldenkrais's particular interest was working with people with infantile neurological disorders, such as cerebral palsy, and other neuromuscular dysfunctions. Classes or private sessions often include people with chronic pain, injury traumas (especially back pain), strokes, and paralysis. Other disorders that may be addressed by the Method include bone spurs, damaged spinal disks, congenital illnesses, physical problems with emotional sources, scoliosis, and learning disabilities.

The Feldenkrais Method also has improved performance skills for actors, athletes, dancers, and musicians. Normal, healthy people take classes to mantain or improve a balanced and happy lifestyle. Do remember, however, that individuals with certain conditions, such as serious orthopedic and neurological ailments, have specific challenges that would be more effectively addressed in private, Functional Integration sessions. Talk to your Feldenkrais instructor to determine the best kinds of sessions for you.

READ MORE ABOUT IT

THE FELDENKRAIS METHOD

Awareness Through Movement: Health Exercises for Personal Growth
by Moshe Feldenkrais
(New York: Harper & Row, 1972/1977)

The Potent Self: A Guide to Spontaneity
by Moshe Feldenkrais and Michaeleen Kimmey
(San Francisco: Harper & Row, 1985)

*Body and Mature Behavior: A Study of Anxiety, Sex, Gravitation and
    Learning*
by Moshe Feldenkrais
(New York: International University Press, 1949)

RESOURCES

The Feldenkrais Guild
8718 West 110th Street, Suite 140
Overland Park, KS 66210
(913) 345-1141

- ❑ practitioner list
- ❑ publications
- ❑ trainings

The Institute for Movement Studies
721 The Alameda
Berkeley, CA 94707
(415) 254-6558
- ❑ information
- ❑ classes
- ❑ trainings

Healers

What Are the Different Kinds of Healers?

There are many kinds of healers: people trained in esoteric knowledge, those possessed by the spirit of a dead person, individuals adept at channeling a special quality of energy, and/or persons drawing on the power of a faith. The Western traditions of healing are wide-ranging and have many labels:

- ❏ Absent Healing
- ❏ Clairvoyant Diagnosis
- ❏ Energy Healing
- ❏ Faith Healing
- ❏ Magnetic Healing
- ❏ Laying-On of Hands
- ❏ Psychic Healing
- ❏ Psychic Surgery
- ❏ Spiritual Healing
- ❏ Spiritist Healing

Healers in each of the categories draw on the help of powers or beings from another realm or reality. Whether invoking the grace of God or clairvoyant knowledge, these women and men gain knowledge through initiation or trial, by a long apprenticeship training, or after some accident, illness, or near-death experience.

These healers can spend years not only developing specific techniques but also taking rigorous moral or spiritual trainings in order to manage well the powers available to them. The more legitimate healers are known by word of mouth, not by their advertisements.

History and Development of Psychic Healing

Despite the old joke, it is healing that is the oldest profession in the world. It grew out of the tribal shaman/healer tradition. Explorers and anthropologists characterize shamanic healing as involving rituals, plants, and chants. Western history describes its healing traditions in the language of touch and magnetism. Sumerian, Babylonian, Assyrian, and Egyptian stone tablets and papyri depict laying-on of hands, as in the Ebers Papyrus. In the fourth century B.C., the Greek dramatist Aristophanes wrote of witnessing the restoration of sight to a blind man and fertility to a barren woman by a healer's touch at the Asklepian temples.

The Bible records what we now call faith healing. The prayers and touch of the prophet Elijah brought a boy back to life. Jesus raised Lazarus from the dead, restored sight, and healed the lame. So did the Apostles. In fact, healing was an important work in the early Christian church.

As the healing tradition in the church declined, the power of healing was assigned to royalty. "Royal Touch" or "King's Touch" was supposed to have cured such diseases as tuberculosis or scrofula. Shakespeare refers to Edward the Confessor's "healing benediction" in *Macbeth*. Philip I of France and Olaf of Norway were reputed to be successful healers.

In medieval and Renaissance Europe, many widows and elderly women acted as healers in the shaman/herbal tradition, until the Inquisition labeled their work witchcraft. The religious fathers nearly wiped out Europe's shamanic heritage. The West is left with only its fragments, such as herbal medicine, imagery, music therapy, and healing.

With the growing split in Western belief between body and soul, faith and logic, science reigned as the new method of organizing thought. Early scientists tried to discover the mechanism for healing to explain the phenomenon in logical, scientific terms.

One of the first modern physicians, Paracelsus, conceptualized a sympathetic system of medicine. His theory was that the magnetic forces of the heavenly bodies influenced humans through subtle emanation or fluid. This magnetic vital force radiated within and around the body—a notion akin to the concept of aura.

Franz Mesmer, the father of hypnotism, called this subtle energy "fluidum" and "animal magnetism." His patients were made to hold "bacquets," iron rods charged with healer-treated water, during treatment. In the 1780s, Mesmer's healings were ascribed to imagination or hypnotism and he was discredited. However, his work echoes in some twentieth-century experiments, and several researchers vindicated Mesmer in the 1960s.

Dr. Bernard Grad at McGill University in Montreal worked with a modern healer, Oscar Estebany. Grad ascertained that healing energy could indeed be transferred to water, confirming Mesmer's theory and work. He also showed that this healing energy could stimulate plant growth rate and accelerate the healing of wounds in rats.

A researcher in Atlanta, Georgia, confirmed Grad's work and also demonstrated the effectiveness of distant or absent healing. Famous healers Olga and Ambrose Worrall accelerated the growth of rye grass from 600 miles away, using visualization and prayer.

A nun and biochemist at the Human Dimensions Institute at Rosary Hill College, Dr. Justa Smith, also worked with Estebany. Dr. Smith discovered that high intensity magnetic fields accelerate chemical enzyme reactions. The longer Estebany held a test tube, the more rapid was the enzyme reaction rate. She also found that healers could repair damaged enzymes. This demonstrated that healing energy could counteract a natural entropic—or disordering—trend. But while the scientists struggled to isolate the mechanism of healing, real healing was taking place outside the laboratories.

Spiritist healers in the Philippines and Brazil sparked much interest in psychic surgery in the '70s and '80s. One healer, Dr. Adolf Fritz, a late World War I German physician, "operates" through a Brazilian doctor, Edson de Quiroz. First channeled through a simple mechanic, Ze Arigo, Fritz chose to communicate through a licensed physician after Arigo's death in an auto accident, perhaps to avoid the legal hassles Arigo/Fritz suffered from the Brazilian Medical Association.

On the other side of the world, Poland licenses several medically supervised bioenergy healers. In 1982, Mietek Wirkus was certified by the Communist government's panel of scientists, with the blessings of the Polish Catholic Church, to use his energy-channeling gifts to facilitate the work of conventional medicine.

Now practicing in the United States, Wirkus conducts workshops and trainings, and encourages further research in paranormal healing.

Research psychologist and author Dr. Lawrence LeShan also offers trainings. Believing that healing can be taught, he studied successful healers, such as the Worralls, Kathryn Kuhlman, and Agnes Sanford, to create a method to teach others healing techniques.

Some holistic pioneers have worked with healers in creating widely accepted theories and techniques. Dolores Kreiger, for example, a nurse and university teacher, developed her research with Estebany and other healers into Therapeutic Touch. History having come full circle from the ancient practice of healing through touch, nurses trained in TT effect positive changes by "laying-on of hands," or by nearly touching their patients while working with the individual's energy field. Therapeutic Touch is now taught in hospital, nursing, and university programs.

Unfortunately, all the encouraging news of these esoteric arts returning to civilized consciousness is balanced by some sobering discoveries in the past two decades. Scientists and skeptics have helped expose fraud in some healing businesses.

Cure tours to the Philippines, taken by scared and desperate patients, were popular in the 1970s. However, the popularity ended quickly after a worried husband obtained a sample of the cancer tumor a healer alledgedly cut from his wife's body and had it analyzed. The supposed tumor turned out to be animal guts.

How Do Psychic or Other Healings Work?

The main difference between native shamanic healers and faith or psychic healers is touch. Psychic healing usually, but not always, entails laying-on of hands. Healers sometimes use other parts of their bodies or just touch the subject's aura or energy field. Shamanic healers tend to use ritual, symbols, and psychology, rather than direct contact with their subjects. However, since our Western healing tradition grew out of the original tribal practices, there are some parallels in tools and approach.

The elements of healing detailed by psychologist Stanley Krippner, from his research on shamanic and psychic healers in South America, can be applied to all realms of healing—psychic and allopathic included. They are:

❏ Shared world view: The naming of the illness relieves the patient, who then feels that the healer understands what is going on with him.

❏ Healer's personality: The subject perceives some "inner force" possessed by the healer that appears to be therapeutic.

❏ Expectant faith: The subject's confidence is induced by the healer's reputation, created atmosphere, and healing paraphernalia.

❏ Technique: Specific mechanisms for healing are used. Krippner's list ranges from medicine and exercise to shock- and group-therapy, but technique can also apply to magnetic energy and use of symbols or talismans.

Krippner tells the story of a "painless surgeon" who operates on his fellow South Americans. They never wince. But some affluent Americans who seek him out for a cure "scream bloody murder." The natives "know" this surgeon is painless, while the Americans don't, so for them the rusty knife hurts! It's the power of belief systems. And we Americans usually assign our faith to our indigenous healers, the MD's.

Scientists are working hard to explain miracles such as Lourdes, the success of spiritual healers like Kathryn Kuhlman, the possibility of channeling "bioenergy," or the mechanism of laying-on of hands. While Grad's and Smith's experiments demonstrated some magnetic influence in healing, it took researchers until the '80s to create an ultrasensitive machine that could prove it. The Superconducting Quantum Interference Device (SQUID) can detect a small but measurable increase in the magnetic field emissions from some healers' hands during healing.

The continuing Therapeutic Touch studies focus on detecting increased hemoglobin, which is popular as a physiological index of healing activity in the subject's body. Hemoglobin carries oxygen, literally the breath of life for cells.

However, the most consistent explanation from healers themselves is that they support, catalyze, or help build the subject's own healing energy or mechanisms. Whether it is the spirit working with the faith healer awakening some inner will to live, the bioenergy of the therapist transmitting and balancing energy to a diseased organ, or the psychic surgeon's operation treating the subject's etheric body, patients ultimately heal themselves.

Applications and Cautions

People seek out healers to treat almost any kind of ailment or disease. They are often desperate. Conventional medicine is not working (cancer is a common disease brought to all types of healers). Or they are very religious and believe in the power of faith.

In Poland, Mietek Wirkus has worked on people with autoimmune and inflammatory diseases, helping to relieve the pain of arthritis. He eliminates energy blocks and disturbances that contribute to headaches, back pain, migraines, and psychological traumas. One internist sent him a man suffering from insomnia, indigestion, chronic fatigue, and depression. A single session with Wirkus cleared all symptoms. The Polish healer says, however, that there are some conditions that consume too much energy, and with which he cannot work, such as schizophrenia and multiple sclerosis.

Greg Schelkun, a Marin County, California, healer who draws his power from the Christian faith, says he and his spirit helpers invoke the healing spirits of his clients to help with such diverse conditions as cancer, diabetes, and AIDS. Schelkun sees the source of all illness as spiritual problems—in his view, "the face of their God has changed." Healing is regaining that connection to God or faith or their own inner wisdoms.

In his work, Schelkun says he talks to the spirit of the illness, learning what lessons the symptoms are trying to present. Whether his healing is addressed directly in those terms or just at the level of spirit and aura, Schelkun works to bring his clients in touch with themselves, to tap into their inherent healing abilities.

While I had decided that faith or psychic healing was one of the modalities I would not try for myself, I realized after my interview with Schelkun that healers don't have to use touch to transmit healing energies. His ideas, words, and presence during our conversation had sent waves of energy through me. I felt palpably charged with a new perspective that was not just intellectual. It was in my heart. If I ever feel in crisis about any illness, physical or otherwise, I know that I would turn to him to help restart my own healing drive and energy.

For many health consumers, the real benefits of these healing arts may be out of reach. We, after all, do not live in the cultural context of the shaman. Our culture does not encourage belief in the power of the spiritualist. Nor, and this is important, does it train us to sort out the huckster from the true inspired healer. More than in any other medical or healing art, I think the phrase *caveat emptor* —"let the buyer beware"—applies here.

READ MORE ABOUT IT

HEALERS

Healing States: A Journey into the World of Spirit Healing & Shamanism by Alberto Villoldo, Ph.D. and Stanley Krippner, Ph.D.
(New York: Simon & Schuster, 1986)

Realms of Healing
by Stanley Krippner and Alberto Villoldo
(Millbrae, CA: Celestial Arts, 1976)

Spiritual Aspects of the Healing Arts
edited by Dora Kunz
(Wheaton, IL: The Theosophical Publishing House, 1985)

Healing the Divine Art
by Manly P. Hall
(Los Angeles: The Philosophical Research Society, 1978)

The Folk Healer: The Mexican-American Tradition of Curanderismo
by Eliseo Torres
(Kingsville, TX: Nieves Press, 1984)

Occult Medicine Can Save Your Life: A Modern Doctor Looks at Unconventional Healing
by C. Norman Shealy, M.D.
(Columbus, OH: Brindabella Books, 1975/1985)

RESOURCES

Association for Research and Enlightenment, Inc. (A.R.E.)
P. O. Box 595
Virginia Beach, VA 23451
(804) 428-3588
❏ information
❏ membership
❏ publications
❏ conferences

Spiritual Emergency Network (S.E.N.)
Institute for Transpersonal Psychology
250 Oak Grove Avenue
Menlo Park, CA 94025
(415) 327-2776
(returns call collect)

Healing Light Center
204 East Wilson Avenue
Glendale, CA 91206
(818) 244-8607
❏ classes
❏ research
❏ consultations

American Society for Psychical Research, Inc.
5 West 73rd Street
New York, NY 10023
(212) 799-5050
❏ information
❏ publications
❏ classes

Herbalism

What Are Herbal Medicine and Herbal Remedies?

Herbal Medicine is the use of any plant part—leaf, seed, stem, flowers, root, bark—for the relief of certain complaints, conditions, or ailments. Herbs are valued for savory or aromatic qualities as well as medicinal use. Technically, fruits and vegetables can be included in this kitchen medicine chest, too.

History and Development of Herbalism

The history of herbal medicine is the history of every culture which turned to local flora for food and medicine. Humans have used plants to heal since the first cavewoman gathered vegetation to feed her family, flavor the food, and heal her children. As the earliest known form of medicine, knowledge of specific plants' curative powers was passed down from generation to generation in the family and tribe.

Eventually, the role of healer expanded to include shamans, or priest/healers. Herbs were used in healing rituals and religious ceremonies. The Hebrew Passover meal includes the ritual of eating horseradish to symbolize the bitterness of life. Records from ancient Egypt to the Middle Ages reveal herbal medicine mixed with faith healing and magic. The *kahunas,* Hawaiian medicine people, still use native, tropical plants for shamanic medicine rituals that predate recorded history. Some historians attribute the burning of midwives as witches to their use of herbs for "magic," including birth control and abortion.

Modern medicine traces its roots back to the Greek philosopher Hippocrates, who wrote about plant remedies, as did the second-century Greek physician, Galen. In the early 1800s, Samuel Thomson, a self-taught doctor in America, patented compounds of plant medicine which he learned from the Indians. Patented medicines became very popular and the Shakers became the first to grow herbs in large quantities to meet a growing demand. While the vogue of "patented medicines" eventually gave rise to cure frauds and the belief that herbal medicines are nothing more than "snake oil," Thomson was an important source for contemporary writers who recorded much of what we know about nineteenth-century Native American Indian herbal lore.

This century's discoveries of modern drugs, such as digitalis, curare, cocaine, and quinine, are based on native herbal wisdom. However, in the early 1900s, the economics of the new, mass manufactured drug therapies overshadowed the use of herbs and natural substances. The allopathic physicians and their use of drugs (treating disease with agents to produce different effects) were becoming the healers in modern societies.

Herbalism continues to be a mainstay of many societies, as folk medicine is intimately tied to the natural environment in which we all live.

"Remember, its original name was 'The Art of Simpling'— simple medicines for simple people from simple plants," says Savita, a Marin County, California, herbalist who lived for many years in the Bavarian Alps learning European folk medicine. "The art is learning how to *receive* from nature." Savita coauthored a book in Germany that included herbal wisdom and herbal home remedies. Germany has a 400-year-old tradition of health practitioners, sanctioned by law, who rely mainly on herbal remedies in their treatment of patients. "Every spring, the country people, the *volk*, go into the woods to pick seasonal plants to make a spring soup. These are the herbs that help cleanse the blood and energize the system," she adds. "The ingredients are there for them to use. Where you are has what you need."

Many parts of the world still rely on local vegetation as their medicine chests. Researchers in the fields of medical anthropology and ethnopharmacology continue to turn to these "simple folks" to study the use of plants as medicine. Scientists explore the curative powers of native plants, hoping to distill their active ingredients into modern drugs.

Interest in the self-healing power of herbs is growing in America, too. Herbal teas, once in the domain of health food stores, are now stocked at the local supermarket, used both as a substitute for coffee and as home remedies. Modern mothers are beginning to use peppermint teas to settle bad stomachs, just as their grandmothers did.

How Do Herbal Medicines Work?

Herbal medicine is central to healing in every traditional culture from India's Ayurveda and China's Traditional Chinese Medicine to Native American medicine and Anglo-American folk medicine. Herbs in all these cultural traditions are used to cleanse, heal, and nourish.

Herbal medicines are said to work biochemically, triggering neurochemical responses in the body. Taken in moderate doses for long enough, these biochemical responses become automatic, even after one stops taking the herbs. Herbal formulas have three basic functions:

❏ Elimination and detoxification: Herbs are used as diuretics, laxatives, and blood purifiers—one step in healing.

❏ Health management and maintenance: Herbs are used to counteract physical symptoms and stimulate the body's own self-healing powers.

❏ Health building: Herbs are used to tone the organs and nourish the tissues and blood.

Herbs such as fennel, cayenne, psyllium seeds, and licorice stimulate the circulatory, digestive, nervous, and eliminative systems in the body and strengthen its ability to cleanse itself. Edema (or bloating) from excess waste material in body cells can occur from too much or the wrong kinds of foods, or from white cells attacking bacteria or viruses but not being eliminated. In a sluggish body, the lymph system—the body's cleansing and garbage disposal mechanism—does not push out the inactive refuse. Herbs can help speed up elimination in the blood, lymph glands, and intestines.

Healing herbs have been found to contain alkaloids. Alkaloids are basic substances from which some modern drugs, such as morphine and quinine, are synthesized. Native Americans chew the inner bark of willow trees for headaches. Willow is high in salicylic acid, the active ingredient of aspirin. European folk medicine has long recommended foxglove for "dropsy," the fluid accumulation from heart, kidney, and liver dysfunction. An English country doctor, William Withering, isolated the digitalis in foxglove, and digitalis is still used as an active ingredient in heart medication.

Herbs, plants, fruits, and vegetables are nature's storehouse of nutrients. Particular herbs and plants, such as papaya, seaweed, and some kinds of sprouts have concentrated amounts of easily assimilable nutrients for the normal growth and functioning of both body and mind. Then there are the toning or tonic herbs, plant parts that sustain the body's resistance to aging and stress factors. Red clover, bee pollen, and wheat grass invigorate the blood. Parsley juice is good for the gallbladder, spleen, and kidneys; dandelion root, for the pancreas and liver. Taken regularly, tonic herbs help us better withstand the typical stresses of modern lifestyles.

Laboratory analysis has confirmed much folk wisdom. Papaya has long been used for bad digestion. Science has since isolated different digestive enzymes and one of them, papain, is plentiful in unripe papaya. Dandelion root is high in minerals and is used to treat anemia. Seaweeds like kelp and dulse are rich in vitamins and minerals and make excellent food supplements.

How Are Herbs Used?

The holistic health movement has sparked new interest in traditional medicines which still use herbs and plants as curative tools. Most homeopathic remedies are plant-based. Naturopathy incorporates herbs and plants into its wide variety of nature cures, as does folk medicine. Iridologists also tend to be nutritionists and herbalists, recommending plant remedies for organic stress patterns read in the eyes. Aromatherapy typically prescribes inhaling essential oils of plants in steambaths. Bach Flowers and other flower essence remedies represent the subtle energy branch of herbalism, infusing the plant's healing power into spring water via sunlight.

There are many systems for using herbs. English herbalists tend to use single herbs for a specific ailment or condition, though they often combine them into compounds. The Chinese make their herbal prescriptions in carefully formulated combinations to achieve more general effects and benefits. Ayurvedic medical practitioners put their herbs in the pungent curries of India's everyday food.

Some people don't have the patience to boil up the strange-smelling Chinese herbal medicine, says Savita. Americans have "McHerb, the fast-food herb—single herbs in capsules you buy off the store shelf," she points out.

Herbalists create herbal formulas for many different types of applications. The form depends on the circumstances, condition treated (internal or external), type or part of the plant, and the person to be treated. While our "fast-food herbs" are the most convenient, there are many ways to use herbal remedies:

- ☐ Ointments, salves, lotions, and oils, in which the herbal properties are infused into oil.

- ☐ Tisane, in which various parts of plants are brewed into a tea.

- ☐ Decoctions, in which the herbs are boiled down into a thick concentrate and strained.

- ☐ Infusion, in which more delicate herbs are steeped in boiled water.

- ☐ Mastication, in which bark, roots, or leaves are chewed.

- ☐ Inhalation, in which steamed or atomized fluids are breathed in.

- ☐ Capsules/Tablets, which are taken by mouth for the herbals to be absorbed through the GI tract.

- ☐ Herbal extraction drops, which are held under the tongue where they are absorbed quickly through sublingual mucous tissues.

- ☐ Douches or enemas, in which herbal extracts wash or are absorbed by the vaginal or intestinal walls.

- ☐ Rectal or vaginal suppositories, which draw out toxins or treat infections, swellings, cysts, or hemorrhoids.

- ☐ Herbal baths, in which absorption takes place through skin pores or lungs via steam.

- ☐ Tinctures/Liniments, in which herbal essences are infused in alcohol.

❑ Poultices, in which leaves, juice, and roots are ground or crushed and then applied to the skin; or in which the plant parts are heated, soaked, or boiled, then mixed and applied to the body in plasters.

❑ Syrups, in which the herb's essence is extracted and preserved in glycerides (sugars).

Applications and Cautions

Herbs can be slow-acting, gentle medicinals, and an alternative or complementary treatment for chronic conditions like allergies. Regularly eating local honey, taking bee pollen, or chewing honeycomb is a common folk remedy to inoculate against hayfever, for example. Chilies in Latin American cooking and tumeric in East Indian dishes can help clean out amoebas from the intestines.

"In countries where it's not safe to drink the water, eat their local spices," advises Savita.

There are fast-acting herbs, too. A friend of mine always has an aloe plant in her kitchen in case of cuts and burns. Sometimes she trims her dog's nails too short and uses aloe to coagulate the blood.

There are many books that describe herbs and list their many applications. Remember that what works for 99 people may not for the 100th, and that person may be you. Test small amounts and pay attenton to any change in how you look or feel. There are many healing plants that also have toxic qualities. Stick with those that have no toxic properties unless you are under the care of a professional herbalist whom you have checked out and trust.

While cultivated herbs may not be as potent as wild herbs that have survived and thrived in nature, you should know what you are buying. If you pick your own herbs in the wild, start with a guide. Not all plants are gentle and harmless, and in cultures that still rely on herbal medicine, the herbalist spends a long time learning. The difference between healing and poisonous plants or beneficial and harmful applications can be subtle; a mistake, fatal.

READ MORE ABOUT IT

HERBALISM

The Way of Herbs
by Michael Tierra
(New York: Washington Square Press, 1983)

Natural Healing with Herbs
by Humbert Santillo, B.S., M.H.
(Prescott Valley, AZ: Holm Press, 1984)

Herbal Medicine: The Natural Way to Get Well and Stay Well
by Dian Dincin
(New York: Gramercy Publishing, 1979)

Culpeper's Herbal Remedies
by Dr. Nicholas Culpeper
(North Hollywood: Wilshire Book, 1977 ed.)

Jeanne Rose's Herbal Body Book
by Jeanne Rose
(New York: Perigee Books, 1976)

Using Plants for Healing
by Nelson Coon
(Emmaus, PA: Rodale Press, 1963/1979)

RESOURCES

American Herb Association
P.O. Box 353
Rescue, CA 95672
❏ information
❏ directory of product resources
❏ membership
❏ newsletter

California School of Herbal Studies
P.O. Box 39
Forestville, CA 95436
(707) 887-7457
❏ classes
❏ certification

Herbal Studies Course/Jeanne Rose
219 Carl Street
San Francisco, CA 94117
❑ information (SASE)
❑ correspondence course

East West Herbology
P.O. Box 712
Santa Cruz, CA 95061
(408) 429-8066
❑ publication
❑ correspondence course
❑ workshops

Homeopathy

What Is Homeopathy?

Homeopathy is a system of medicine based on the principles of "like cures like" and "less is more." A term coined by its German founder, homeopathy comes from the Greek *homois* and *pathos,* meaning "similar sickness." Agents that cause the symptoms of sickness in a healthy person can cure the cause of those same symptoms in an unhealthy person when used in extreme dilution. The homeopathic preparations or remedies are essences of naturally occurring substances derived from plants, animal materials, and natural chemicals.

History and Development of Homeopathy

Samuel Hahnemann, the founder of homeopathy, was born in southern Germany in 1755. Qualified as a physician by the time he was 24, Hahnemann became disenchanted with the rather crude medical practices of the time—bloodletting, purgation, and suppression of symptoms. A linguist and student of botany, Hahnemann quit his practice to work as a medical translator. While translating a standard medical text, *Materia Medica,* he read a reference to quinine. The Scottish physician William Cullen said that the plant cured malaria because of its bitter and astringent qualities. Reasoning that there were other bitter, astringent plants that didn't cure malaria, Hahnemann began taking quinine to investigate for himself its curative powers.

He came down with malaria's intermittent feverlike symptoms—cold extremities, drowsiness, flushed cheeks, and thirst—but without the shivering fever itself. Hahnemann felt he had discovered "similars," which he thought Hippocrates had originally referred to in his 4th century B.C. writings.

161

Both the Father of Medicine and another important figure in modern medicine, Swiss physician, philosopher, and alchemist Paracelsus (1493–1541), emphasized the use of "similars"—substances that make one ill but can also cure, in small enough doses. Hippocrates recommended treating vomiting with emetics (agents that cause vomiting); Paracelsus is reputed to have successfully treated victims of the 1534 plague with "pills" made of bread and minute, pinhead-sized amounts of the patients' excreta. Hahnemann's work confirmed this principle, which is now called the Law of Similars, or "like cures like."

Hahnemann continued to experiment with a long list of materials, recording the effects they elicited. Infused in alcohol, some material tinctures seemed too strong, causing toxic effects in a few patients. He experimented with diluted tinctures, discovering that dilution not only eliminated toxic effects but also increased the remedy's power, scope, and depth of action.

In 1810, Hahnemann published his findings and philosophy in *The Organon of the Healing Art,* which laid the foundation for the practice of homeopathy. In 1821, he published a long list of proven remedies in *Pure Materia Medica* and *Chronic Disease.* Homeopathic practice began to spread throughout Europe and arrived in America in 1825. Homeopathic treatment is mentioned in accounts of the 1832 cholera epidemic in Europe, as well as of later epidemics of scarlet fever, dysentery, and yellow fever.

Homeopathy became quite popular durng the mid-1800s, especially with the intelligensia. Mark Twain, Louisa May Alcott, Horace Greeley, Daniel Webster, and Henry Wadsworth Longfellow are among the historical figures who supported homeopathy. In 1844, prominent homeopathic physicians in New York, Boston, and Philadelphia formed America's first medical association, the American Institute of Homeopathy, which predated the American Medical Association (AMA) by several years.

While Europe hummed along with allopathic (today's conventional drug medicine) and homeopathic medicines coexisting as healing systems, the AMA turned its professional back on homeopathy in America. Like osteopathy and chiropractic, the AMA first tried to co-opt this other medical system. Doctors who studied or practiced homeopathic medicine were barred from joining the AMA. Later, the Association's Code of Ethics was revised to admit homeopaths.

In 1911, the Flexner Report, an influential evaluation of

medical schools, panned homeopathic training programs, which then lost their federal and private funding support. Homeopathy faded into the quiet corners of America, practiced by a small minority of lay and allopathic physicians.

Homeopathy flourished in Europe, however. The British royal family is still treated by a homeopathic physician, Dr. Ronald Davey. Queen Elizabeth II is said to travel always with a homeopathic first aid kit. By 1977, the United Kingdom had six homeopathic hospitals in its National Health Service; they served more than 86,000 people in their outpatient clinics.

British pharmacies dispense homeopathic prescriptions along with drug prescriptions. Elsewhere, South Africa officially recognized homeopathy in the '70s. Homeopaths are also popular in Italy, France, Germany, Brazil, Argentina, and India. Mahatma Gandhi was a supporter of homeopathy.

In the United States, homeopathy as a medical practice is done under the license of one of the other accepted forms of medicine—so a homeopath must also have qualified for a chiropractic, oesteopathic, or acupuncture license, or be an M.D. The current resurgence of interest in homeopathy in America includes allopathically-trained doctors. Some estimates say that about half the homeopathic doctors are also medical doctors. But suspicion and competition still exist.

In 1983, a medical doctor in Arizona had his license to practice medicine revoked by the local medical board for including homeopathy in his treatment consultations. His successful fight for reinstatement led to the establishment of the Arizona Board of Homeopathic Medical Examiners in 1986, placing homeopathy on an equal status with allopathy. In Arizona, however, homeopaths must first be M.D.s or osteopaths before adding homeopathic training to their qualifications.

While the AMA no longer has an official position against homeopathy, the California Medical Association lists homeopathy as quackery along with hair analysis, Laetrile, naturopathy, clinical ecology, and megavitamin therapy.

How Does Homeopathy Work?

Homeopathic philosophy is based on the belief that symptoms are signs of the body's effort to throw off disease; one must treat the whole person, not the symptoms. Homeopaths seek to strengthen the body's own ability to heal itself, believing the body can cope with most chronic and acute illnesses. Homeopaths not only recognize modern technical medicine as better suited to treat emergency conditions requiring heroic measures or mechanical diseases requiring surgery, but also work side by side with other medical systems.

One basic distinction between allopathic and homeopathic medicines is the view of symptoms as signs indicating a disease pattern, not the disease itself. The word *symptom* is from a Greek root word meaning "falls together with something else." Homeopaths see symptoms, such as fever, diarrhea, or coughing, as adaptive responses by the body in defense of itself; signals of something else going on. Allopathic doctors tend to see the symptom *as* the problem.

Research by physiologist Matthew Kluger and a team at the University of Michigan Medical School has shown that the body prepared itself to fight infection by creating a fever. Fever helps increase the mobility and activity of white blood cells, the body's storm troopers against disease. It also enhances production of interferon, a body-produced chemical which can be effective against viruses. Diarrhea expedites the dumping of pathogens or irritants from the colon; a cough clears breathing passages. Fever, diarrhea, and coughing are not the disease, only the sign of an internal problem and the body's action to solve it.

While fever should be lowered when it is high enough to cause serious damage to the individual's health, modern medicine's tendency to suppress many symptoms is, in the homeopathic view, like shutting up the person who yells "help" from the window of a burning building. The homeopath wants to know where is the fire? Why is this person calling for help with these symptoms? The perceived problem of the victim may be a sign of an underlying pattern, a deep-seated disharmony which is the source of the distress.

At the heart of homeopathic doctrine and treatment are Hahnemann's three principles: Law of Similars, Single Remedy, and Minimal Dose.

The Law of Similars means that substances that cause a disease or symptom in large amounts will cure the same condition in minute amounts. Like treats like. Allopathy, today's medicine, tends to treat by "contrary" substances, using agents that produce different or opposite effects. We take aspirin to kill the pain of a headache, not asking what the pain is trying to tell us.

Single Remedy means using the one substance that most closely models the symptom of the disease, and therefore is most effective to counterbalance the condition. Modern medicine may use several drugs in a single treatment, with one drug prescribed to counterbalance the potentially toxic side effects of another. Homeopathy says one substance can mimic the entire symptomology annd treat the underlying cause.

A headache is different in experience for each person, with a different location, duration, kind of pain, and varous factors which make it worse or better, and accompanying symptoms. Some people get dizzy. Others feel nauseous, or get a sore throat or rash. These are all clues to both the individual's constitutional type and the nature and source of the pain. The homeopath selects one of a myriad of remedies for a headache depending on her in-depth investigation of the symptoms.

When a remedy is selected, the homeopath chooses the appropriate potentiation or dilution for treatment, the Minimal Dose. Homeopathic remedies are tinctures of natural substance diluted so many times that, at 24x potency (10–24), none of the original substance can be found in the alcohol or water mixture. The more it is diluted, the deeper-acting the remedy.

How does the remedy work if there is little or no substance left in it? Most homeopaths will admit that they don't exactly know. They seem content that they get results without knowing the specific mechanism. Many homeopaths talk about remedies "resonating" with the client's "vital force"—the same life force call *chi* in Chinese medicine and *prana* in Indian Ayurvedic medicine.

Homeopathic "vital force" echoes a growing view that the body or whole human being is a bioenergy system. Several writers have proposed explanations in more scientific terms for how remedies work.

Each person is a dynamic entity, vibrating on both a bodily and a cellular level at a certain energetic frequency. A healthy person oscillates at a more harmonious frequency than an unhealthy one, whose imbalance in vibration reflects a cellular imbalance. The right remedy is a booster shot of subtle energy, returning the cellular bioenergetic system to its proper vibrational frequency. If the body-being is "in tune"—resonating at its proper rate—the immune system cells can throw off the toxins of illness.

Remedies with a low concentration of substance vibrate with

a unique, high intrinsic energy state. The tincture is not active in the molecular, chemical sense, like a drug, but is imprinted with an energy pattern transferred by the potentiation process, the increase of the energetic power of the remedy. Further, these energy patterns are thought to be self-replicating in bioenergetic systems, like the body. In other words, the remedy transfers its energetic imprint to the body's fluids or cells, which then spread the new resonation throughout the body, transforming other cells.

If the wrong remedy is taken, it misses the "center of gravity" of the disturbance—a frequency miss—and nothing is supposed to happen. According to Dr. Richard Gerber in his landmark book, *Vibrational Medicine,* the principle of resonance dictates that a biological system will only accept certain resonant frequencies. The remedy has to be an exact match in order to stimulate movement to a new level of energetic organization and function.

What Happens in a Homeopathic Consultation?

Like most medical systems, the first session with a homeopath is longer in order to take a detailed personal history. The doctor will ask questions about domestic, personal, psychological, and medical aspects of the illness or complaint. For example, she or he may ask about one's attitude toward life, history of illnesses, temperature, likes and dislikes in food, weather, drink, people, preference for solitude or crowds, relationships and sexual appetite, or how one sleeps at night.

The fact that I often woke up with my arms thrown above my head was significant in determining a remedy. Such details are important. Exactly similar symptoms of disease still call for different remedies for different people, because the constitutional type or the total picture of the person varies. The detailed history helps determine the particular remedy.

Homeopathy as a medical system is both a science and an art. The doctor selects a remedy and its potency through a combination of scientific deduction and intuitive insight. The homeopath must have a talent for observing and the ability to glean information on a whole list of variables and then remember salient points of a long list of remedies in order to choose the one remedy to use.

The client or patient is sent home to take the single-dose

prescription, and waits usually four to six weeks before the next consultation. Be prepared for a healing process with several stages. The remedy may peel away the first layer of symptoms, revealing another set of symptoms or "center of gravity" of the condition to be addressed. Your condition may change or improve to the extent that more of the same or another remedy is required to keep the process going.

Hering's Law of Cures says: "Cure proceeds from above downward, from within outward, from the most important organs to the least important organs, and in the reverse order of appearance of symptoms." This means that the body will deal with symptoms and causes, starting with the most distressing or most central to the disease. The "center of gravity" or focus of the distress can shift to the next most distressing condition, etc. For example, the primary symptom may move from a stomach ache to a skin rash—from within outward—indicating progress in the Law of Cures.

World-renowned homeopath and teacher George Vithoulkas says that while the first evaluaton is the most important for the homeopath, the follow-up appointments are the most difficult. Here is where the long-term experience and observation skills, as well as critical thinking and analysis, of a doctor pays off. Is the client truly improving? Is the aggravation of symptoms a sign of healing? Is the change of symptoms the exposure of a next layer of healing?

Chosen correctly, a remedy will often stimulate a healing crisis, the temporary aggravation of symptoms. This is a good sign, as long as the aggravation isn't too severe. A healing crisis may be intense, but never life threatening, my homeopath reminds me.

Once a change in symptoms or a healing crisis indicates the body has marshalled its defenses to throw off the disease, the doctor waits and has you observe your symptoms and progress. The healing crisis, like a vaccination reaction, is an encouraging sign that the remedy, like the shot, is working. The process relies on the correct reporting of symptoms by the client and the insight and skills of the doctor.

Applications and Cautions

Homeopathy is appropriate for most reversible illnesses, chronic or acute. Modern technical medicine is the best for emergency or mechanical dysfunctions, or severely acute situations. Homeopathy doesn't set bones, repair hernias, or remove burst appendixes. The danger of acute peritonitis (massive infection of the abdomen) from appendicitis demands heroic allopathic measures, such as surgery.

However, homeopathic remedies are ideal complementary or secondary treatments for these and other traumas. Arnica or Bach's Rescue Remedy administered in the ambulance on the way to the hospital can help reduce shock. Other remedies taken after an operation can support the recovery period. Remember, the essential action of homeopathic remedies is to strengthen the body's own healing powers, treating the whole person, not just the disease.

Homeopathic authors recommend homeopathy for:

❑ Chronic problems: colitis, peptic ulcer, high blood pressure, and obesity while still in the reversible, not acute stages.

❑ Mild deficiencies: anemia, hormonal imbalances, nutrient assimilation. Treatments help enhance the body's ability to make or metabolize substances and strengthen the immune system.

❑ Allergies: especially hay-fever, migraines, allergic rhinitis, eczema, or to food and environmental substances. Again, remedies strengthen the body and its immune system to deal with the problem.

❑ Some infections: e.g., bladder, bronchitis, asthma, sore throat, pneumonia, otitis (middle ear infection).

❑ Prevention: to counterbalance genetic or environmental predisposition to common disease by the general strengthening of a constitutional remedy; to help prevent severe bruising and discoloration prior to activities of potential trauma or after surgery; to prevent miscarriage and postpartum blues.

The cautions and contraindications revolve around the severity of the condition and the weakness of the patient. Overwhelming infections, such as peritonitis and meningitis, require swift action with antibiotics to prevent permanent physical damage. Similarly, highly infectious diseases, such as typhoid, cholera, and smallpox, call for antibiotic treatment to prevent epidemics.

The elderly, who are in weakened condition, need antibiotics for acute viral attacks, such as pneumonia. However, homeopathy can play an important supporting role in the convalescent phases of all these treatments when the conditions are no longer life threatening.

There are different types of homeopaths. Classical homeopaths stick with one remedy. This is the science and the art in its purest form. It requires a depth of experience—literally, practice—to be really good at it.

Some modern homeopaths practice isopathy, acute medicine or Western medicine's symptom suppression. They may prescribe remedies for particular diseases rather than treating the whole person. Buying remedies at the health food store is another fast-food version of a traditional healing system, the laypersons' isopathic use of store-bought remedies. These commercial products are panoramic formulas. Each little pill or bottle of drops contains essences of several remedies indicated for the specific symptom on the label. Hopefully, one of them will hit the mark.

Then there are eclectic homeopaths who combine their craft with other healing arts. Vitamin therapy, nutrition, and chiropractic are popular complementary practices. My first homeopath used a German machine to measure the bioenergetic flow in my Chinese acupuncture meridians. He also administered the constitutional remedy in a vitamin B shot. Classical homeopaths view this trend as muddying the waters for diagnosis and treatment. Using other healing modalities may cloud the overall picture of symptoms by relieving some of them; a true picture of the person and the healing process cannot emerge, obscuring the constitutional type of the client.

Remember, there is no licensing, per se, for homeopaths. Check for training and state certification under one of the other medical care systems licensed in your state, if the homeopath chooses to practice that form of medicine also.

The best news is that some conceptual barriers are coming down in the minds of traditional allopathic doctors. In England, a homeopath is on staff at a medical school under a fellowship for Complementary Medicine. In America, some M.D.s are training as homeopaths. With the best of both worlds to choose from, these physicians can offer both types of remedies: the speedy intervention of allopathy's drugs and surgery and the holistic nurturance of homeopathy.

READ MORE ABOUT IT

HOMEOPATHY

Homeopathy: Medicine for the 21st Century
by Dana Ullman
(Berkeley: North Atlantic Books, 1988)

Homeopathic Science and Modern Medicine
by Harris L. Coulter, Ph.D.
(Richmond, CA: North Atlantic Books, 1981)

Everybody's Guide to Homeopathic Medicines
by Stephen Cummings and Dana Ullman
(Los Angeles: J. P. Tarcher, 1984)

Psyche and Substance: Essays on Homeopathy in the Light of Jungian Psychology
by Edward C. Whitmont
(Richmond, CA: North Atlantic Books, 1980)

The Healing Art of Homeopathy: The Organon of Samuel Hahnemann
edited by Edward Hamlyn, M.D.
(New Canaan, CT: Keats Publishing, 1979)

Bioenergetic Medicines East and West: Acupuncture and Homeopathy
by Clark A. Manning and Louis Vanrenen
(Berkeley: North Atlantic Books, 1988)

The Science of Homeopathy
by George Vithoulkas
(New York: Grove Press, 1980)

RESOURCES

National Center for Homeopathy
1500 Massachusetts Avenue N.W., Suite 42
Washington, DC 20005
(202) 223-6182
- ❏ information
- ❏ publications
- ❏ directory
- ❏ conferences
- ❏ products
- ❏ classes

Homeopathic Educational Services
2124 Kittridge Street
Berkeley, CA 94704
(800) 359-9051
(415) 653-9270
- ❏ information
- ❏ products
- ❏ publications
- ❏ speakers

International Foundation for Homeopathy
2366 East Lake Avenue, East Suite 301
Seattle, WA 98102
(206) 324-8230
- ❏ information
- ❏ publications
- ❏ seminars
- ❏ research
- ❏ referrals (directory)
- ❏ speakers
- ❏ membership

Hypnosis And Hypnotherapy

What Are Hypnosis and Hypnotherapy?

While the scientific and therapeutic literature is filled with discussions of just what hypnosis is and how it works, researchers in the field describe hypnosis as the inducing of a trancelike state of heightened suggestibility or compliance. It is a state of consciousness or awareness that is not sleep but not an awake state, either.

Before the nineteenth century, subjects induced into this trance state were labeled "somnambules" or sleepwalkers. That name described the sense that the hypnotized person is half-asleep and responding to only a narrow range of stimuli in a rather automatic way. In the mid-1800s, a British surgeon coined the term *hypnosis* from the Greek *hypnos,* or "sleep." It's half right.

The hypnotic state is somewhere between waking and sleeping states. Electroencephalography (EEG) shows brain rhythm that is neither a waking nor sleeping pattern. Some researchers question whether this special quality of attention is more focused or more mobile than normal, but they agree that the subject's orientation to external reality is diminished.

Beyond the laboratory tests and definitions are the range of natural spontaneous hypnotic states. Daydreaming is a stepping stone on a continuum of altered states. Spacing out while driving along very familiar routes, being mesmerized by a white line ("highway hypnosis"), or "going unconscious" are light hypnagogic states. The deep relaxation during a particularly effective massage where you "go away" but don't fall asleep is another example of a hypnagogic state.

Terrified, disoriented, starving, or extremely ill people may go into spontaneous, self-protective hypnotic states. The narrowed range of response to stimuli shields them from some physical or emotional pain or focuses their senses on survival behavior. Sometimes it can focus attention and energy to accomplish a normally impossible task, such as a mother lifting a car off her child.

In recent years, a growing number of psychotherapists have been choosing hypnosis as a therapeutic tool. Some trained hypnotists are beginning to practice hypnotherapy. The difference between hypnosis and hypnotherapy is the quality of interaction between the expert and client.

Holly Holmes, Director of the Hypnosis Clearing House, a well established training center in the San Francisco Bay Area, says hypnotherapy gives the individual more control and the opportunity to go deeper into the physical and emotional roots of problems than in psychotherapy. The distinction, she says, is the degree of client participation and volition.

"Hypnosis is the use of suggestion. The client passively receives ideas or instructions from the hypnotist," she says. The hypnotist is an authority figure telling you your nicotine craving is gone or your hunger will be satisfied with less food. Hypnotherapy is therapy under hypnosis. Therapy is the process of discovery and recovery from psychoemotional traumas that affect the productive living of life.

"Hypnotherapy focuses on the underlying need to smoke or eat. The relationship between the hypnotherapist and client is more interactive, less suggestive. The techniques work whether one is hypnotized or not because the therapeutic techniques work. The hypnotic trance, however, allows the therapy to work on a deeper, more primal level."

Holmes believes that hypnosis enables the client to work on a deeper, more effective level, accessing information not only from the subconscious but also from the higher consciousness or Higher Self (see Past Life Therapy).

History and Development of Hypnosis

The use of hypnotic states to heal goes back to the early eras of human history. Preliterate cultures used drumming, chanting, and dancing to induce altered states. These were healing rituals for both the community spirit and sick individuals. The Druids called hypnosis "magic sleep." The Greeks and Egyptians had "sleep temples" for healing. Patients were given curative suggestions while they were in a trance or slept. Modern hypnosis and hypnotherapy traces its beginnings to Franz Anton Mesmer, an eighteenth-century Austrian physician who demonstrated cures using "animal magnetism" (later, *mesmerism*). His theatrical approach alienated his medical contemporaries, who convened a commission to investigate his claims. They denounced him as a charlatan in 1784. Mesmerism fell into disrepute, ignored and left to isolated doctors who continued to explore this phenomenon on their own.

Hypnosis has had its ups and downs on the way to acceptability. In the 1820s, a dentist extracted the first tooth and a woman delivered the first baby in painless childbirth using only a trance state for anesthesia. However, in the 1840s, the British medical establishment censured physicians for using hypnosis as anesthesia. James Esdaile, a Scottish surgeon, reduced the common surgical mortality rate (50 percent in those days because surgeons washed their hands only *after* the operation) to 5 percent using hypnosis. He also washed his hands—the factor that made the most difference. His colleagues were suspicious. John Elliotson resigned as head of staff at the University of London's hospital, under pressures for his use of hypnosis.

It was Dr. James Braid who finally gave hypnosis its modern name and modern induction techniques. He introduced the use of eye fixation and verbal suggestion for engaging the subject's concentration. By the 1880s, there were two schools of thought on this new medical tool that was once again the object of investigation, especially in France. The Nancy school saw hypnosis as a hysterical state showing some abnormality in the nervous system. The Salpêtriere group, headed by Jean-Martin Charcot, saw hypnosis as a normal phenomenon, attributing its power to the influence of suggestion. History has proven Charcot right as far as he went.

Again, hypnosis was due for more bumps on its rocky road to credibility. Freud studied and translated works of both of the French groups. Not particularly skilled at induction, he dropped hypnosis from his developing field of psychoanalysis, thus cooling interest in hypnosis for a generation of therapitsts. Military doctors used hypnosis to treat shell shock and battle fatigue after both world wars, but it was still regarded as a fringe technique. Finally, the British Medical Association convened an investigating committee and in 1955 approved hypnosis as a valuable tool. The AMA followed suit three years later.

Since then, the scientific community has published volumes of research, trying to dissect and explain just how hypnosis works. And, despite the intellectual controversy, hypnotherapy is today taught at medical schools and is recognized as a tool for healing and changing behavior. The theoretical thinking and research in hypnosis spawned several other therapies, including Autogenic Training and certain relaxation techniques (see those chapters).

How Does Hypnosis Work?

Most experts say hypnosis is a distinct state of consciousness on the continuum of brain states between awake and deep sleep. A few scientists have put forth the theory that the hypnotized subject is playing a role, rather than being in an altered state. They say it is like getting caught up in the emotion of a play on stage so you feel a part of it, identify with it. Some hypnotists will tell resistant or unskilled clients to "act as if" they were hypnotized as a way of inducing the trance state.

As a state of consciousness, the subject experiences distinct phenomena. One is "trance logic," the suspension of normal critical analysis, allowing a tolerance for logical inconsistencies. Trance logic opens the subject to responding to suggestion. A man given a pencil to hold who is then told that it is a hot metal rod will drop the pencil as if it is burning his hand. If asked later whether he saw a rod or a pencil, he would state that he saw the pencil but experienced the heat.

Examples of this kind of phenomena led to one of the hot debates about hypnosis. Is the change experienced real or perceived under hypnosis? For example, the hypnotist suggests to subjects that they are deaf. Do trance subjects truly not hear or do they only think they cannot hear?

Research demonstrates that the body and body chemistry change in trance states. In one experiment, a girl could hold her hand in a bucket of ice water for only 30 seconds in normal consciousness. Blood levels of cortisol, a measure of stress response, were high. Under hypnosis, she could hold her hand in the water for 30 minutes with no rise in blood cortisol levels.

In age regression experiments, foot reflexes changed. Stroke the sole of the foot of infants before the age of six months, and the reflex movement of the big toe is up; after six months, the toe moves down. In adults regressed under hypnosis to age six months or younger, their toes reflex up in the infant reaction. How does that happen? What is going on in the body-mind of the hypnotized subject? Nobody can quite explain.

While not everyone is easy to hypnotize, anyone who is motivated and approached appropriately can learn to go into a trance. The average hypnotist will find 5 percent of her clients unresponsive. About 45 percent can only enter a light hypnotic state on the first try and another 35 percent are able to reach a medium level of trance. The remaining 15 percent are able to let go and experience the deeper trance states on a first induction. Medical hypnotists and hypnotherapists use deep trance states for anesthesia and posthypnotic suggestion. These are the states where the subject can lose all sensation of pain, be compliant, and very receptive to suggestion.

There are many myths and misconceptions about hypnosis. Often a hypnotherapist must ask what clients think hypnosis is and reeducate them so they are able to relax and allow themselves to enter trance states. The blocks to being hypnotized include:

❑ Fear of loss of control: not trusting one's ability to censor inappropriate suggestions or to wake oneself if necessary.

❑ Previous bad experience: an insensitive hypnotism experience or a spontaneous hypnotic state during a frightening circumstance.

❑ Unconscious resistance: based on unrecognized fears or misconceptions about hypnotic states.

❑ Mismatch of hypnotist and subject: personality clash or a lack of rapport.

❑ Attitude of hypnotist: the motivation for the induction doesn't feel right and the subject knows it consciously or unconsciously.

Generally, the more intelligent and creative people are, the more responsive they are because they understand they can control and use hypnosis for their own benefit. Imagination and the ability to concentrate are two important traits in good hypnosis subjects. It is easier to hypnotize a willing subject but not impossible to work with a skeptic, especially if his imagination and concentration are engaged.

According to Holly Holmes, there are three ways to measure whether you are hypnotized:

❏ Trance phenomena: observable physical changes

❏ Subjective experience: perceptual changes

❏ Rapport with hypnotist: cooperative interaction, a blending of energies; perhaps, at times, a telepathic connection

External evidence of a trance state is observed when:

❏ Body becomes very still, limbs heavy

❏ Eyelids flicker with rapid eye movement (REM), as when dreaming

❏ Eyeballs roll up as when asleep, or look bloodshot

❏ Eyes tear at corners

❏ Pupils dilate

❏ Speech pattern or voice changes

❏ Body movements become jerky or automatic

Internal or subjective evidence of being hypnotized can range from feeling a special sense of connectedness with the hypnotist to achieving selective awareness, becoming more focused. The special rapport with your "guide" can be a deep trust which can include an increased responsiveness to suggestion. A narrowed span of attention shuts out unnecessary or distracting sounds, thoughts, or sensations to help you focus on the purpose of the hypnotic session.

Applications and Cautions

There are four main applications of hypnosis: entertainment, memory recall, medical treatment, and skill enhancement or personal growth.

Stage hypnotists, popular at fairs and conventions, are entertainers who work with volunteers on stage. They ask embarrassing questions or plant posthypnotic suggestions, such as to kiss the first good-looking man the subject sees. They also can make certain subjects so rigid that they can be suspended, like planks, between two chairs.

While the trance lowers resistance to the authoritative guidance of the hypnotist or "operator," most experts agree that the hypnotized person or "subject" will not do anything that is against his moral or self-preservation instincts. People embarrassed during stage hypnotism allow themselves to be embarrassed.

My first hypnotic experience was a stage performance. Highly responsive, I keeled over at the flick of the hypnotist's finger (into the arms of his assistant), a standard test. But when he asked me to do something very embarrassing, I felt myself come out of the trance quickly, as if I were arriving at the top floor on a fast elevator. I looked him in the eye and said, "No, thank you." He quickly moved on to the next person and I was whisked offstage.

These entertainers have done much both to advertise hypnotism's power and to give it a bad name. I felt upset after that stage hypnotism. While the hypnotist's assistant asked if I was okay and offered to talk with me about what happened, the experience brought up feelings I could not understand on my own at the time. I felt too vulnerable to trust a stranger (the assistant) and too overwhelmed by the star power of the hypnotist to say I needed help. Years later, when I tried hypnotherapy, I realized this was a much safer environment for me to experience hypnosis. There is a law against using anyone under 21 for stage demonstrations in England. I would approach casual stage hypnosis with much caution.

Some police departments in the U.S. use hypnotic memory recall to help witnesses remember details of a crime they might not remember under normal circumstances. The LAPD was one of the first to institute trainings for its officers. The British, however, are reluctant to use this techique; the Bobbies are concerned that suggestions made to a witness under hypnosis might prejudice a case in court.

Medical and psychotherapeutic applications continue to develop beyond the early focus on surgical or dental anesthesia and psychological conditions due to anxiety and hysteria. Habit control is a big industry today. Smokers and overeaters have turned to hypnosis to help control their addictions; oftentimes it has worked. While hypnosis has not been an effective treatment for addiction to drugs and alcohol, it has provided addicts with effective adjunct treatment for building self-esteem and reenforcing recovery behavior.

Patients with psychosomatic conditions, such as skin disorders, headaches, migraine, and ulcerative colitis, often find hypnotherapy helpful. Some people with certain types of asthmas, hypertension, and anorexia have been responsive to hypnotherapy. The key is discovering and healing emotional issues underlying the dysfunction of a biological system. The Simmonton Imagery Process for cancer patients is an example of hypnosis or self-hypnosis marshalling immune system power to help fight a disease.

Healing in hypnotherapy often comes through interpreting the metaphor of the illness or pain. One woman living the "superwoman" life—a new home, family, work, and husband all demanding her time and energy—tried everything for the pain in her shoulder. Medical, chiropractic, and orthopedic treatments did not help. Massage gave only temporary relief. Under hypnosis with a therapist her "higher consciousness" said the weight on her shoulder was an excuse to take time for herself, such as for a massage. This client made an agreement to take time for herself so that her shoulder did not have to hurt to remind her, and the pain disappeared as she kept that agreement.

Psychosexual disorders usually respond to hypnotherapy, as do bed-wetting, muscle spasms, and chronic pain. Hypnosis can also be effective in increasing resistance to infection and reducing inflammation.

Athletes and businesspeople use hypnosis and self-hypnosis for personal and professional growth. Coaches teach their athletes imagery exercises to help them overcome obstacles to optimum performance. Mental rehearsing, visualization, and exercises to overcome anxiety or poor attitudes are all techniques included in the wider definition of hypnosis. So are creativity techniques that seek to enhance playfulness, attentiveness, relaxation, receptivity, and concentration in trainings for executives, artists, and other professionals.

A warning: Hypnosis is like a gun; it's not the tool itself but the operator who makes it dangerous. Dr. Milton Erickson, one of the world's leading authorities, warns that while hypnosis itself has never caused anyone harm, like drugs and other treatments, people can misuse it.

It is a question of who can handle or control the experience of this altered state of consciousness. A hypnotist should be competent in determining whether someone is too deeply depressed, suicidal, or on the verge of a nervous breakdown, in which case hypnosis might tip them further down that pathological road.

In most states, there is no certification or licensure requirement for hypnotists or hypnotherapists. Make sure that you choose a trained hypnotist, someone certified by a state-approved school of hypnosis.

When determining whether to work with a hypnotist or a hypnotherapist, first ask yourself what you want—a quick fix for a surface problem or a deeper exploration of underlying causes for your condition? Do you want to be told what to do or discover your own inner resources for changing your life? Smoking can be a physical addiction to nicotine that may be overcome with posthypnotic suggestions to help get you through quitting cold turkey. It can also be a sign of some deeper, more powerful and pervasive need that drives you psychoemotionally to suck on a cigarette and fill your lungs with smoke. That deeper need can eventually overpower a posthypnotic proscription against smoking or drive you towards another, equally self-destructive compulsion. As you may guess, I favor hypnotherapy over hypnosis.

Other red flags about hypnosis include becoming too dependent on the hypnotist. Hypnosis, like psychotherapy, is a vulnerable state for the client and can lead to feelings of dependency. The integrity and competency of the hypnotist is vital. Most hypnotists and hypnotherapists teach clients self-hypnosis, empowering them to carry on their own healing processes.

Hypnosis is not the answer for every problem, nor the best approach for some. When doing age regression, it may not be appropriate to either the client or the goal at hand to go back. I have used hypnosis as a shortcut to look at a deeply buried memory. Once uncovered, however, it was too painful to handle on my own and I needed to go back to my old therapist to understand the overwhelming emotions unearthed by my attempt at a quick fix. Often the Higher Self will know not to delve into a particular incident and ignore the guide's suggestion. Sometimes, the guide needs to ask. Again, it is a question of rapport between subject and hypnotist and the intention or motivation of the client.

Finally, pick a thorough hypnotist. The operator may forget to remove a posthypnotic suggestion, cluttering up your life.

Even though the subconscious will eventually reject such mental refuse, it is debatable how long it will take.

READ MORE ABOUT IT

HYPNOSIS AND HYPNOTHERAPY

Hypnosis: Developments in Research and New Perspectives
edited by Erika Fromm and Ronald E. Shor
(New York: Aldine Publishing, 1979)

Hypnosis with Friends and Lovers
by Freda Morris
(New York: Harper & Row, 1979)

The Complete Guide to Hypnosis
by Leslie LeCron
(New York: Barnes & Noble, 1973)

RESOURCES

International Medical & Dental Hypnotherapy Association
4110 Edgeland, Suite 800
Royal Oak, MI 48073
(313) 549-5594
　　　or
11824 Lyon Road
Delta Vancouver, British Columbia
V4E 2S9 Canada
(604) 597-4264
❑ publication
❑ referrals
❑ membership
❑ certification
❑ networking

Iridology

 ## What Is Iris Diagnosis or Iridology?

Iridology is a form of reflexology, a study of how signs of the health of the body and its organs are reflected in the eye. Naturopaths and other health practitioners analyze the iris of the eye for indications of genetic and functional weakness throughout the body. The process is also sometimes called Iriscopy, Iridiagnosis and Iris diagnosis. Fiber patterns, changes in color, and abnormal markings give indications of the body's tissue condition and a client's psychoemotional behavior patterns. The iridologist analyzes his readings of these determinants to form a picture of the whole person, and to ascertain the client's physiological and psychological states.

Iridology uses "eye maps," charts showing parts and qualities of the eye that reveal information about the body's condition. European and American "eye maps" are physiologically oriented. Another kind, the Rayid Model, developed in the 1970s and 1980s, identifies psychoemotional and soul development indicators in the eye to help clients understand themselves and their relationships.

History and Development of Iridology

Like most Western healing arts, iris diagnosis literature cites Hippocrates as an original practitioner. Its early history also includes trainings in iris diagnosis at the Medical School of Salerno. A 1670 book, *Chiromatica Medica,* notes that signs in the iris indicate diseases. Author Philippus Meyens believed that the condition of the heart and spleen could be read in the left iris, the liver in the right. And, on a nonscientific level, people have always looked into the eyes of their fellow humans—and other animals—to determine feelings and physical well-being. Shepherds, for example, have long examined their sheep's eyes to cull the weak ones from the flock.

The mythical origin of modern iridology credits a Hungarian physician, Dr. Ignatiz von Peckzely. As a boy struggling with a captured owl, Peckzely broke its leg. He noticed a dark spot appear just then in its eye. This incident was supposed to have inspired Peckzely to pursue his study of injuries and iris marks as a medical student and surgical intern.

After several decades of comparative study, he developed an iris topology. Superimposing a clock face over drawings of the eyes, he mapped organs across zones identified by hours and minutes. In 1881, Peckzely published his theories in *Discoveries in the Field of Natural Science and Medicine: Instruction in the Study of Diagnosis from the Eye.*

Soon after, Swedish doctor Nils Lilinquist added his observations on color changes. He was the first to identify the effects of drugs, such as iodine and quinine, on the iris. One of his students, Dr. Henry Lahn, brought the practice of iridology to America near the turn of the century. A naturopath and chiropractor, Bernard Jensen has been America's foremost proponent of iridology. He is currently setting up a research center, creating a computerized eye bank, analyzing the irises of hundreds of heart and kidney patients. Each case is catalogued with its correlating iris signs information; Jensen hopes this will aid in standardizing iridology interpretations.

How Does Iridology Work?

The eyes contain thousands of nerve fibers, which are extensions of the brain. Eyes start forming early in the fetus. The muscles that dilate and contract the pupils are derived from nerve tissue in the developing embyro. However, nobody really knows how iris color and patterns are formed. They may be purely genetic markings, but other theories suggest an anatomical reflex connection, or an electromagnetic vibratory influence.

Coupled with other diagnostic techniques, eye examinations can actually give a complete profile of a patient's health care needs. The eyes act as an early warning system for constitutional weakness. Congenital lesions, such as gray, ovoid, or spindle shapes in the iris show tendencies toward diseases inherited from the parents.

These marks can also be indicators of early tissue pathology in the development of chronic conditions throughout the body. Iridologists can identify whether an inflammation has reached an acute, subacute, chronic, or destructive (actual organ tissue loss) stage.

The iridologist studies the shape, color, and quality of the iris tissue, as well as structural patterns, flecks of pigment, and minute changes. The entire iris bioarchitecture reflects an individual's constitutional type.

Each gland and organ has its place on the eye map. However, different researchers have slightly different maps or interpretations. All iridologists say color is significant, for example, but disagree on the meaning. According to Jensen, white indicates overstimulation or increased activity. Others say white signs or cloudiness can show an accumulation of unnatural substances, such as uric acid deposits or arteriosclerosis.

Dark spots suggest insufficient activity, and may also show the beginning of inflammatory disease. Clarity indicates healthiness—a "clear-eyed person." Eye coloring also gives clues to whether medications have affected blood and lymph circulation. Density, the grain of the iris structure, gives information on the firmness, vitality, or general tone of body tissues.

European iridologists are more medically oriented than the Americans. Developed mostly by M.D.s, European eye topology grew out of long-term studies confirmed by autopsies. German doctors tracked individual patients in a clinical study for decades, correlating iris sign observations and health conditions.

The American medical profession has not been so accepting. Studies published in the AMA and American Optometric Association journals showed iris diagnosis to be ineffective. Several iridologists were asked to identify people with abnormal kidney functions from slides of the eyes of 143 patients. The results were dismal, though some evaluators noted poor quality photography.

On the other hand, the University of Rochester and the National Heart, Lung and Blood Institute reported better results. The latter study tracked 8,825 men and women for eight years. Its study showed that visible yellow or gray-tinted white rings around the cornea indeed may alert patients to heart disease risk.

What Happens in a Session?

A "reading" may be part of a visit to your doctor, naturo-path, chiropractor, or nutritionist. However, iridology is growing in popularity as a separate assessment system for many different kinds of practitioners. It may be one of several tools for the typical composite practitioner who combines nutrition or herbol-ogy, a form of bodywork, and a psychospiritual training.

The iridologist usually takes a picture of your eyes as a record and to help you see what he is talking about in the analysis. Or he shines a little flashlight into first one and then the other eye and records what he sees on a chart. Each practitioner has his own style, looking at different aspects of the eye for the information sought. What he looks at depends on whether a general picture of health is needed or an indication of a specific physiological issue. Depending on his primary health care train-ing, the iridologist follows the reading with advice on preventive or supportive health practices, usually nutritional or herbal.

I first met iridologist Jeff Bruno at San Francisco's Whole Life Expo. He was finishing a Clinical Psychology Ph.D. thesis on iris typing and personality measures. Skeptical after reading several books on iridology, I was still curious about possible correlations between personal history, physical health, and the markings in an iris and asked him to do an analysis for me. Jeff's reading impressed me deeply.

I had specific questions about my constitution and stressed digestive system. He saw the colon area in my eye clearer than normal, indicating I had made good lifestyle changes, but needed to take better care of my stomach. He was very gentle in talking about physical and emotional stress indicators.

Trained in the Rayid system as well as being a student of both the American and European eye charts, he was quite com-prehensive in his comments. He made physiological observations and then added wisdom about the possible psychoemotional connections to my condition. He then showed me herbal digestive products and talked about the stomach's dual role in both nour-ishing and nurturing oneself.

Surprisingly, he saw a switch from right- to left-brain domi-nance in my early childhood. In fact, a rigid school system forced me to abandon a left-handed tendency and write right-handed, which exercises the left brain. He also correctly indentified an occasional frustration with speaking, an affect of a slight dyslexia, from markings at the top of my iris. Using the Rayid model, he offered an analysis about my relationships and my soul development challenges—the lessons in life—that was startlingly accurate.

Application and Cautions

Designed as an assessment tool, iridology is used to put together a representative picture of the client. Iridologists study the eyes for indications of nutritional deficiencies, nervous disorders, congested organs, and under- or overactive glands. Iridologists schooled in the Rayid system add observations of emotional signs. These are particularly helpful in understanding psychosomatic origins of chronic or stress conditions.

Like most holistic practices, iridology focuses on preventative measures and constitutonal health-building, rather than specific symptom cures. The eyes give clues to congenital weakness. Knowing the sources of stress or the parts of the body that are particularly affected by stress can help the client change his attitudes and lifestyle for better health.

Books on iridiagnosis list eye traits that are connected to specific conditions, such as stressed liver, kidney, and adrenals. Chapters also cover injury, heart conditions, and anemia, and explain the clues the iris gives about circulatory problems, colon ailments, and possible stages of inflammatory diseases such as arthritis.

I even had one iridologist look at the top of my eyeball and tell me I would fare better as a vegetarian.

If you are going to try studying your own irises, use some common sense. Eyes are delicate organs, sensitive to light. Be careful about the brightness of the light and about how long you shine it into those baby blues, hazels, grays, or browns.

Many iridologists write for the layperson. Each book has its own perspective and interpretations of signs. The charts and handy laminated maps, some with psychological as well as physical trait indicators, do not all agree. Take your findings with a grain of salt or take your eyes (and body) to an expert.

READ MORE ABOUT IT

IRIDOLOGY

What the Eye Reveals: An Introduction to the Rayid Method of Iris Interpretation
by Denny Johnson
(Goleta, CA: Rayid Publications, 1984)

Fundamental Basis of Irisdiagnosis
by Theodor Kriege
(Romford, Essex: L.N. Fowler & Company, 1969)

Iridology: How the Eyes Reveal Your Health and Personality
by Dorothy Hall
(New Canaan, CT: Keats Publishing, 1980)

The Science and Practice of Iridology
by Bernard Jensen, D.C., N.D.
(Provo, UT: BiWorld Publishers, 1952)

Iridiagnosis: Diagnosis from the Eyes
by Victor S. Davidson, N.D., D.O., D.C.
(Wellingborough, Northhamptonshire: Thorsons Publishing Group, 1979)

Iridology: A Patient's Guide
by James and Sheelagh Colton
(Wellingborough, Northhamptonshire, Thorsons Publishing Group, 1988)

RESOURCES

The National Iridology Research Association (NIRA)
P.O. Box 179
Laguna Beach, CA 92652
(714) 494-5342
❏ information
❏ publication
❏ classes
❏ membership
❏ certification

Rayid International
408 Dixon Road—SASR
Boulder, CO 80302
(303) 444-4218
❏ information
❏ publications
❏ referrals
❏ seminars and classes
❏ speakers

Massage

What Are Swedish Massage and Other Massage Therapies?

Massage is a systematic, therapeutic stroking and kneading of the body. The word comes from both the Greek *masso,* to knead, and the Arabic *mass,* to press gently. Therapeutic masseurs and masseuses usually use oil, and the client or patient is unclothed and draped with sheets or towels.

The term *massage* is sometimes used interchangeably with words such as *bodywork, body therapies,* and *body manipulation.* Technically, there are different types of body therapies. Manipulation therapies focus on restructuring the body. These range from Osteopathy and Chiropractic to the Alexander Technique, Rolfing, and Postural Integration.

Bodywork is a catch-all term. Practitioners usually employ it for non-massage systems and techniques that do not specifically adjust or restructure by manipulation, or involve stroking or kneading soft tissue and muscles. The term *body therapy* seems to be used to communicate a therapeutic or healing intent of the system, modality, or session. Energy-based body therapies, such as Acupuncture or Reflexology, emphasize free-flowing vital force, or *chi.* These types of bodyworks apply pressure to the body, but are not strictly massage.

Massage is a healing art that is sensual. When practiced between lovers, it can be sexual. Unfortunately, massage is often misunderstood, and has suffered a negative connotation from a mistaken connection to prostitution. Many masseuses and masseurs use the term *massage therapy* to distinguish their healing arts services from "massage parlor" practices.

There are many styles of massage, many names from which to choose. The following are samples form the wide-ranging kinds of massage available today:

189

❑ Swedish: the original health spa and sports club massage; uses a set routine of basic strokes to work over the whole body.

❑ Esalen: a blend of Eastern and Western approaches, primarily Swedish and acupressure; stresses empathy, communication, and nurturance above the technique.

❑ Organ or Lymphatic Drain: encompasses several styles; focuses on stimulating internal organs such as the liver, kidney, or colon, to flush toxins and mucus.

❑ Lomi: based on a Hawaiian Kahuna tradition; works deep tissue.

❑ Amma: based on ancient Oriental traditions that gave birth to shiatsu and Kahuna energy-based massage; works *tsubos,* or energy points, stroking away from the heart.

❑ Subtle Touch: infuses touch with inspiration; reaches into muscle tension to contact and melt away painful emotional holdings.

❑ Sports massage: used as part of athletic training; focuses specifically on muscle recovery rate to alleviate the aches and pains of exertion and competition.

❑ Rehabilitate or Medical massage: developed by the medical specialty "physiatry" for post–World War II amputees and other wounded veterans; focuses on relieving pain from neurological problems.

History and Development of Massage

The natural use of hands to comfort and heal is documented in rock carvings, papyrus scrolls, and ancient oral histories starting 15,000 years ago. Early medical traditions include the extensive practice of touch, massage, and manipulative therapies in treatments.

Massage was part of classical Greek medical studies. Greek physicians, such as Galen and Soranus of Ephesus, prescribed massage as part of gynecological treatments. Massage was a regular feature of the Roman bath, an early hydrotherapy. The historian Plutarch noted that Julius Caesar enjoyed regular massages.

According to some historians, early Christian church attitudes toward massage and touching shifted from appreciation of their ceremonial and therapeutic roles to condemnation of their erotic aspects. Healing, especially by laying on of hands, had been important work for early Christians. Later, however, the church regarded the body as the repository for sin, obscuring the healing or comforting pleasure of touch. Massage then went underground until after the Dark Ages.

In the meantime, on the other side of the world, the T'ang dynasty in China (A.D. 618–907) had an Imperial Medical Bureau with a special Department of Massage. In eighth-century Japan, Nara Medical College included massage courses in its curriculum. And throughout the East, it was customary for devotees to "anoint with oil" the feet of their guru. Massaging a teacher's feet was (and is) said to transfer special energy or a blessing to the student.

Many families in modern India preserve an ancient tradition of lymphatic massage as a regular health practice. Infants receive a daily massage from birth until they are about three years old. From ages three to six, they are massaged once or twice a week. After six, they are taught to share a massage with family members. Grandchildren play with and give grandparents massages. Wives minister to husbands. Massage is an integral part of family life.

In the West, massage resurfaced in the medical profession at the end of the Renaissance, when Ambroise Pare and other sixteenth-century French physicians began exploring the benefits of body manipulation in treatment. Their writings formed the basis for Henri Peter Ling's development of Swedish Massage, the grandmother of modern massage techniques.

Ling, a University of Stockholm student in the early 1800s, wanted to duplicate the benefits of Swedish gymnastics on the massage table. He created kneading, friction, shaking, and stroking movements to imitate the sport's 47 positions and 800 movements for stimulating and relaxing the body. At first, both the Swedish medical establishment and government rejected Ling's system. But popular support and, probably, friends in high places helped him get a license in 1814 to teach the practice of massage.

Ling's concept caught on in Europe. By the mid-1800s masseurs were part of the European health care system, particularly in sports medicine. Georg Groddeck, a pre-Freudian physician, treated mental patients using baths and massage to help them reach below their conscious level of language.

Health care professionals in America took much longer to see the value of massage. Until the mid-1900s, massage was a privilege of the wealthy and well-traveled, who first discovered its benefits at European health spas. Dancers and athletes were really the only others who used massage, until America's cultural horizons widened in the '60s and '70s.

The human potential movement moved from hippie openness in displaying the body to experiments in bodywork. The Esalen Institute, the Big Sur mecca for the newly enlightened, played host to hundreds of new and old forms of healing arts and psychologies. Massage and a growing number of body therapies became part of the new self-awareness, as well as an intellectual movement. "Body language," a new kind of sublingual communication, was gloriously celebrated at Esalen cliffside hot tubs, as it still is today, at any time of the day and night.

Massage is now an integral part of the bodywork movement. People are creating their own styles using variations of the basic Swedish hand movements. Some practitioners mix in Eastern and manipulative techniques, sculpting the session to the client's needs.

Some states, such as California, require professional massage practitioners to earn a certificate from an approved school. A massage certificate qualifies a practitioner's services for medical insurance reimbursement if the client was referred by a primary care provider. Some local governments also require masseurs and masseuses to register with the police, including having their fingerprints taken.

The American Massage Therapy Association, which certifies and promotes massage therapists, has grown from a handful of members in the '40s to more than 5,000 professionals today. State-approved massage schools teach the basics of massage. Graduates who earn their certificates of completion sometimes go on to train in a bodywork system not recognized by the state, practicing this new system under their massage certification.

By the way, when I visited Sweden's largest bodywork school, Axelson's Gymnastiska Institut, I learned that in Sweden, what we know as "Swedish massage" is called "Classical massage."

How Does Massage Work?

Swedish massage and other massage systems use a variety of basic movements. Stroking is constant pressure while the hands glide over skin. It has a sedating or relaxing effect on muscles. Designed to improve circulation and cellular waste removal, compression strokes knead or use friction. Percussion, used on the meaty parts of the body, soothes nerves, tones skin, and affects deeper organs and tissue.

A massage session can sedate or stimulate the body, depending on the nature or style of strokes applied. The different types of strokes or movements include:

- ❏ Effleurge: light stroking, firm and gentle; centripetal effleurage moves toward the heart, stimulating circulation; rotary or spiral effleurage stimulates the smaller blood vessels in the skin.

- ❏ Pétrissage: firm friction stroking, both deep and superficial.

- ❏ Kneading: rhythmic lifting and squeezing of flesh.

- ❏ Tapotement: light hacking, tapping, or clapping over muscles and the fleshy parts of the body.

- ❏ Touch: simple placing or molding of the hand over a part of the body.

- ❏ Vibration: rapid shaking and pulsating, done by hand or with a machine.

- ❏ Brushing: light fingertip contact done slowly and rhythmically to spread general sensations over the body (it can tickle, too); often done as a finishing stroke.

- ❏ Range of Motion: passive exercising by rotating, flexing, and extending body and limbs to mobilize joints and boost secretion of synovial fluids.

- ❏ Nerve compression: exerting firm pressure to relieve knots or pain at nerve points.

Some studies show that massaging the back can heighten sympathetic nervous system activity—increasing blood pressure, pulse, respiration, and skin temperature. Unlike a very hot bath or strenuous exercise, massage can increase blood circulation without taxing the heart. A vigorous massage wakes up your mind and body. Athlete or executive, you are ready to meet the world, aware of your physicality and with reserves of energy.

On the other hand, gentle massaging can stimulate the para-sympathetic nervous system, decreasing the heart rate. Natural defenses and tight muscles generally relax, digestion hums along. The world feels warm and fuzzy and mellow.

Both the release of muscle spasms and the softening of chronic muscle contractions give the veins and tiny capillaries in the blood system a chance to clear out edema, the collection of stagnant tissue fluid. They also allow connective tissue to regulate better its acid-base (pH) balance, water content, and cellular cleansing action. This aids the immune system in doing its partic-ular cleanup job in fighting inflammation, infection, and allergies. White cells on the microscopic battlefield wade through less debris on their way to zapping offending toxins or bacteria.

Massage's cleansing action is particularly beneficial to ath-letes and the weekend jocks who suffer aches and pains after particularly strenuous or violent exercise. Excess lactic acids, coming from glycogens stored in the muscle and liver and burned during exertion, clog the muscles. The body must drain this residue, or convert it to sugar for storage.

On its own, the lymph system may take hours, even days, to complete the cleansing. Left in the muscle, the lactic acid forms tiny crystals that can cause pain and cramping. Massaging soft tissue and muscles speeds up the metabolic reabsorption or release of the fluid toxins.

A classic experiment (done long before animal rights pro-tests) illustrates the power of massage to cleanse muscles and the body. Doctors injected a hind leg of two rabbits with India ink. Over the next month, one animal had its leg massaged, the other didn't.

Both were then killed and dissected in the name of science. The untouched rabbit's leg had an ink stain in its muscle. But the doctors could find no trace of ink in the muscle, or in the entire body, of the massaged rabbit.

One direct benefit of massage for the athlete is improved "recovery rate," the ability for muscles to perform after exertion and rest. In *The New Massage,* his classic book on body condi-tioning, George Inkeles quantifies the effectiveness of various specific techniques in draining fatiguing waste fluids from muscles. For example, five minutes of rest after doing 50 push-ups yields a 20 percent recovery. This means the subject can then manage another 10 push-ups. But by following 50 push-ups with five minutes of Fluid Release massage, the exerciser is capable of doing 37 to 50 more push-ups, up to a 100 percent recovery!

The effects of massage go much deeper than conditioning muscles and cleansing the body. Touch is a human necessity. Anthropologist Ashley Montagu wrote a whole book on the history and meaning of touching. Skin, the organ of touch, with hundreds of nerve reflectors and 15 feet of tiny blood vessels per square inch, is probably the most complex organ in the body after the brain. Every massage movement sends multiple signals throughout the nervous system.

What Happens in a Massage Session?

You can receive a massage at an office, in a health club or spa, at home, or just about anywhere else. It is best to find a quiet room, out of the way of people, away from phones and other interruptions. Most practitioners use a massage table for ease and comfort, though it is not necessary. If taken at a spa, a massage is often accompanied by a sauna, mud bath, soak in the Jacuzzi, or warm blanket wrap.

After you are ushered into a small room, you undress and the masseuse drapes you with a sheet or towel (you should remove your contact lenses as well). If the masseuse doesn't know you, she should ask if you have any pain, or have experienced recent injuries, operations, or illnesses.

Unlike primary health care providers, most massage technicians do not take an extensive health history. Massage therapists may ask a few more questions before starting a massage. This is the time to alert the practitioner to any cautions, areas to avoid, or instructions from your physician.

The massage therapist will often start with the feet, or with a light stroking on the back, to orient you to her touch as you begin to relax on the table. Then, depending on the style of massage, the masseuse strokes, kneads, taps, and presses your flesh into delicious putty.

I have had lots of massages, both formal and informal. The Swedish massage, for example, follows a set formula or routine.

It's popular at health spas and sports centers. Swedish is a good choice for beginners, for those just getting used to bodywork in the nude, for persons who don't want to talk to the masseuse, or for anyone seeking a general toning up.

After I experienced the nurturing and personalized touch of massage therapy and other bodyworks, I found Swedish massage a bit too impersonal and routine for my taste. However, I recently treated myself to two days at the hot springs and mud baths of Calistoga, California. I had not had a Swedish massage in years and wanted to remind myself what it was like.

I discovered that, as with all bodywork, the Swedish experience depends on the masseuse. I had the best massage I can remember there—the masseuse was nurturing, yet she still maintained the impersonal distance taught in the Swedish tradition.

I learned another valuable lesson that weekend about overdoing massage. During trainings, I always heard "moderation in all things." More than three massages a week could be too much for the body. But I never really believed I could overindulge my body.

Wrong! I had scheduled a steambath and Swedish massage, an herbal wrap, an enzyme bath, and an herbal facial—one each morning and afternoon. And each time I got a foot massage. By the fourth foot session, my feet were so tender, they begged to be left alone! I had finally reached bodywork satiation.

Applications and Cautions

A good massage feels terrific. Rubdowns and therapeutic bodywork increase physical stamina, sexual vitality, and foster a general sense of well-being. Done in a gentle, nurturing way, they can take us back to the peace and safety of a mother's arms.

Besides conditioning an athlete's muscles and body, massage can relieve stiffness, pain, and numbness in us ordinary folks. Careful massaging around the joints or an injury can help reduce some swelling in sprains and fractures.

Both Chiropractic and Reflexology talk about the neuroreflexive connection between soft tissue manipulation and effects in other parts of the body. Massage can stimulate digestion or help tone the colon, an internal muscle, to help relieve constipation. Various massage techniques are good for headaches, nervous upset, and insomnia. Some healers and physicians have prescribed massage for conditions as diverse as gout, polio, and obesity.

Midwives throughout history and all over the world administer massage in prenatal and postpartum care. Mothers in labor receive tension-relieving shoulder and back rubs. Massage helps stretch the perineum to prevent tearing as the baby's head emerges from the birth canal. Breast massage stimulates the flow of milk. And baby massage accelerates developmental progress and helps strengthen the constitution of the newborn.

While touch is good for almost everybody, there are a number of contraindications for massage and massage therapies. Exercise caution with large bruises, fever, inflammation, swelling, and skin eruptions. Check with your primary care provider before receiving deep pressure or soft tissue manipulation massages if you have any of the following conditions:

- ❑ Osteoporosis or brittle bones
- ❑ Inflammation or arthritic conditions
- ❑ Hypertension, high blood pressure, or heart condition
- ❑ Varicose veins (avoid massaging both limbs if present on one)
- ❑ Thrombosis (blood clots that cause obstructions in a vessel)
- ❑ Aneurysm (weakness or dilation of an artery)
- ❑ Skin, muscle, or bone diseases
- ❑ Kidney condition
- ❑ Unhealed bone fracture
- ❑ Recently torn ligaments, tendons, or muscles
- ❑ Diabetes
- ❑ Tumors
- ❑ Frostbite
- ❑ Pregnancy

Some of these conditions may actually benefit from an energy-based bodywork, such as Therapeutic Touch. However, most can be adversely affected by increased circulation or metabolism that comes with massage, in some cases possibly spreading the condition to surrounding tissues. Again, your treating physician should approve any kind of massage therapy.

READ MORE ABOUT IT

SWEDISH AND OTHER MASSAGE THERAPIES

The Massage Book
by George Downing
(New York: Random House, 1972/1988)

The Complete Book of Swedish Massage
by Armand Maanum with Herb Montgomery
(New York: Harper & Row, 1985)

Amma: The Ancient Art of Oriental Healing
by Tina Sohn and Donna Finando
(Rochester, VT: Healing Arts Press, 1988)

Unwinding: Super Massage for Stress Control
by Gordon Inkeles
(New York: Weidenfeld and Nicolson, 1988)

Chi Self-Massage: The Taoist Way of Rejuvenation
by Mantak Chai
(Huntington, NY: Healing Tao Books, 1986)

The Book of Massage: The Complete Step-by-Step Guide to Eastern and Western Techniques
by Lucinda Lidell
(New York: Simon & Schuster, 1984)

RESOURCES

American Massage Therapy Association
National Information Office
1130 West North Shore Avenue
Chicago, IL 60626
(312) 761-AMTA (-2682)
❏ information
❏ publications
❏ state contacts for practitioners

❏ membership
❏ certification
❏ research
❏ presentations
❏ schools and trainings referrals

Associated Professional Massage Therapists
1746 Cole Boulevard, Suite 225
Golden, CO 80401-3210
(303) 526-1740
❏ information
❏ publication
❏ directory
❏ membership
❏ speakers
❏ research

Myotherapy

What Is Bonnie Prudden Certified Myotherapy?

Myotherapy is a technique developed by fitness expert Bonnie Prudden for defusing trigger points in muscles. Trigger points are tender or irritable spots in the muscles that can cause pain. They can refer pain as well, sending it to be felt in an entirely different place from the original location. Prudden's Myotherapy is a system of locating and applying pressure on trigger points and exercises to retrain the muscles. The combination relieves acute or chronic pain and helps prevent its return.

History and Development of Myotherapy

While based on ancient principles, this system's history is relatively short. Bonnie Prudden, that energetic physical fitness and exercise authority who helped awaken the U.S.A. to the flabby condition of its children in the '50s, discovered Myotherapy in the '70s. Actually, she took a principle from a standard medical procedure and applied it with her hands. Though the Chinese knew about trigger points 3,000 years ago, a German physiologist, Max Lange, identified them for twentieth-century science.

Dr. Janet Travell researched and documented myofacial (muscle tissue) pain due to trigger points, creating Trigger Point Injection Therapy (TPIT) in the early '40s. She used it to help Senator John F. Kennedy with his debilitating back pain in 1955 and went on to serve as President Kennedy's personal physician in the White House.

Trigger Point Injection Therapy releases excessive muscle contractions or spasms with an injection of a solution of saline

200

and procaine into painful muscle spots. Her therapy includes applying moist heat and coolant spray, and stretching the muscles to give them the message to RELAX!

Prudden had been working with patients referred by Dr. Desmond Tivy, coaching them in corrective exercises after Trigger Point Injection Therapy or an operation. One day in 1976, a woman walked in with a painful stiff neck that set her head to one side. Usually, Prudden would find sore spots, circle the trigger points, pack that person off to Dr. Tivy for injection treatment, and then wait for them to return for muscle re-education. This time, in searching for the trigger point, Prudden pushed a little harder than usual. The woman let out a yelp, but when Prudden let go, the woman's head was straight and the pain was gone.

Prudden had had a similar problem—and solution—in her youth. She was on a mountain climbing trip and woke up with a painful neck that pulled her head to one side. Dr. Hans Kraus, a TPIT practitioner, was part of the group, but had none of his normal equipment on hand. He pressed his thumb into her neck, causing such a pain that Prudden says her knees buckled. But he didn't stop until he had squashed the knot. It worked. Her pain and stiff neck were gone and she could complete the climb. Were these two incidents just flukes?

Prudden's next appointment was with a woman suffering from tennis elbow. Instead of the usual resistance exercises to improve the range of motion, Prudden tried holding all the trigger points she could find. The woman walked out with a full range of motion in both elbow and shoulder. Prudden was excited. She knew she had stumbled onto something.

Reporting her findings to Dr. Travell, Prudden worked out timing in holding trigger points (usually seven seconds). Prudden continued to work with Dr. Tivy, quickly mapping out a system of myotherapy. She eventually established her School and Institute for Physical Fitness and Myotherapy in Massachusetts and published her ground-breaking book *Pain Erasure* in 1980, followed by *Myotherapy* in 1984 and a number of other how-to books. Prudden's Institute trains and certifies Bonnie Prudden Certified Myotherapists℠.

How Does Myotherapy Work?

The term *myotherapy* is really a generic term. *Myo* means muscle, and there are other massage organizations unrelated to Prudden that include the word myotherapy in their names or treatment regimens. What makes her myotherapy unique is its focus on trigger points and her close ties with the medical world in developing the technique. And, unlike general massage practitioners, Bonnie Prudden Certified MyotherapistsSM only take patients referred by medical physicians. This is to ensure that clients are screened for other possible pathologies before trying myotherapy.

While the medical world can't exactly explain how and why trigger points work, it does say that they are highly irritable spots found in abnormally tightened bands of skeletal muscle. Muscles pick up trigger points when they have been "insulted" or damaged. An insult can occur due to many causes, such as an injury suffered in an auto accident, a seemingly harmless slip on the ice, or even our trip down the birth canal.

Trigger points are involved in "armoring," Wilhelm Reich's term for layers of contracted muscles, tightened against physical or emotional pain. Trigger points in armored musculature "fire" in response to physical trauma or emotional stress, setting up spasms that tighten the muscles. They can calm down again after treatments such as chiropractic manipulation, heat, whirlpool, massage, or aspirin, which temporarily chase the pain away. However, according to Prudden, these trigger points lie dormant until internal or external environmental pressures stimulate them to fire again, shooting a message of pain to the brain, setting up another spasm.

Her point is that the various strategies and medical treatments meant to treat the pain will only bring temporary relief. Unless the trigger point is eliminated and the muscle reeducated, it will fire again in response to stress. She claims 95 percent success with myotherapy for immediate and long-term relief.

There are two types of trigger points: Matrix and Satellite. The first seems to be the result of an original insult. Matrix points are primary causes of local and referred pain; a matrix trigger point in the neck can send pain messages to the head. These points can be tricky because the referred pain may hurt more, masking the true source. We might treat the headache but not the sore spots in our neck and shoulder muscles that may be the real or primary sources of the pain. Satellite points spring up near the original problem. These points can set off matrix points. Prudden stresses that erasing some points (such as a matrix point) while overlooking others (such as satellites) may leave little "time bombs" waiting to trigger pain again.

Just what lays down these trigger points in our bodies in the first place? When Prudden is "sleuthing after pain" she takes a client's detailed history—what happened at birth and early childhood, accidents, operations, occupations, and experiences, plus life incidents that might have caused emotional distress—as clues to trigger point locations.

Prudden lists five major causes:

❑ Birth: A baby's colic may really be a headache caused by the firing of trigger points which were created as the baby squeezed down the birth canal. Forceps deliveries and other common bumps and bruises may indicate potential trigger points.

❑ Accidents: Trivial or severe, these injuries are obvious sources of muscle "insult." Those tailbone twinges from a fall or jammed foot muscles from slamming on the brakes could turn into chronic back pain from trigger points.

❑ Sports: Runners, for example, get shin splints (muscles that pull away from the shin bone) and calf muscle spasms. Untreated, shin splints and spasms can refer pain to the knee joint. The knee may be treated but continues to feel sore because the cause is further south.

❑ Jobs and Hobbies: Manual labor is an obvious cause of accidents or strains. However, the limited or repetitive motions of desk-sitters and computer jocks earn them their own aches and pains in the shoulders, neck, back, and legs, especially if they don't exercise.

❑ Disease: Prudden cites her own posttraumatic arthritis from her ski injury as an example. Multiple sclerosis, Epstein-Barr, and lupus are medical conditions that typically generate trigger points, as well as high fevers and seizures. She adds that the noxious products of disease, and even alcohol and drugs, can lay down trigger points as well as fire existing ones.

There are several points to remember about myotherapy and working with trigger points. Prudden, Tivy, and Travell stress that incomplete or improper treatment of trigger points defeats the process and can potentially cause more pain. Any satellite or matrix points missed by the therapist can rekindle old trigger points supposedly inactivated. Massaging trigger points without releasing them may just aggravate the pain.

Travell recognizes that properly applied massage, acupuncture, ultrasound at low intensities, manual compression, acupressure, and shiatsu can be as effective as her Trigger Point Injection Therapy, but that it must be done by a qualified therapist.

Finally, it is not just a question of squashing out those trigger points that feel like knots. Most important is taking care to keep muscles capable of unconscious free movement, as opposed to restricted, protective, armored movement. And fitness booster Prudden provides plenty of exercises in her books to get and keep them in shape.

What Happens in a Session?

After the standard practice of taking a medical history, including details of jobs and hobbies, Cheryl Whitaker put me through a simple muscle function assessment. While I passed with flying colors, she noticed that one shoulder seemed higher than the other. This went along with my complaint about headaches and TMJ (jaw pain and misalignment).

Myotherapy is done on a table. She started working on my back, finding some real tender spots on my buttocks about where they sew on the back pockets. She said these trigger points related to numerous sporting accidents and my shoulder-head pain. Just as the book says, she worked away from the primary problem area, loosening up surrounding muscles that helped release my shoulder and neck points once she got there.

I was prepared for torture; she was gentle but firm. She pushed into the sore points to the point of pain, easing off a little if I said it was too much.

I had *so many* sore points relating to my head pain. And many seemed to be hidden in ignored parts of my body (like under my armpit and below my collarbone), requiring lots of knowledgeable attention.

After working on a zone, she would knead the area and then put it through some passive stretching exercises. These exercises became part of my "homework" to retain the newly-created flexibility. The stretches are one of the keys to myotherapy. As Whitaker says, you might as well not do myotherapy if you are not going to follow up with the exercises.

As suggested, I brought a friend with me to the appointment to learn how to work on me. It was fun and reassuring to have a friend with me who knows where to push on many of the knots that Whitaker found on me. However, it's not a reflection on my friend Tracy, but the treatment is done better—more appropriately and completely—by a certified practitioner.

The pain can be exhausting but the release and the subsequent relief are worth it. And I *can* do the "Quick Fix" points on myself when life tensions or deadline pressures trigger my patterned headache.

Applications and Cautions

Thanks to Prudden's energetic and easy-to-read explanation of the system in her books, just about anyone can understand and use her myotherapy. *Myotherapy's* "Quick Fix" section is a kind of owner's manual. It outlines myotherapy's extensive system of trigger points, pressure, and exercises to reclaim the body's innate flexibility and freedom, what Prudden calls "Pain-Free Living."

She divides the body into five zones with seventeen segments. For example, Zone I is "the headache zone," with five segments. Myotherapy works trigger points related to the many types of headaches and migraines, tinnitus (ringing ears), TMJ (a painful jaw condition), stuffy nose, and tic douloureux. Pain can be referred between segments—an old head injury can make the teeth or jaw ache. Zone V covers feet and legs, where pain from shin splints can refer down to misaligned metatarsals or up to knee pain and backaches.

She even includes a handy guide to the muscle strains, insults, and trigger points typical of a long list of sports. The Quick Fix is first aid for on-the-spot pain. However, all this potential self-help information is only one message of Prudden's books. A permanent fix is possible.

When chronic pain has become unbearable, or expectations for a pain-free life are high enough to motivate a serious treatment program, Prudden details her pain-erasure campaign. The exercises are more extensive, the trigger point pressure more detailed, and the sessions needed more numerous.

Dr. Tivy summarizes who might try myotherapy for chronic or recurring pain. People with:

❑ Head, neck, torso, or limb pain due to functional problems; structural problems like slipped disks or broken bones are precluded.

❑ A structural problem controlled as well as possible (e.g., arthritis controlled by medication) but who still suffer functional pain.

❑ Structural problems that may be treated by surgery (e.g., suspected lumbar disk prolapse). Trying myotherapy may make the difference in avoiding surgery.

Tivy says those with problems better treated by medication or surgery or those who bruise easily (the anticoagulated) should not try myotherapy. And remember, it is *painful;* one needs to be pretty motivated to go the full course.

READ MORE ABOUT IT

MYOTHERAPY

Myotherapy
by Bonnie Prudden
(New York: Ballantine Books, 1987)

Myotherapy: Bonnie Prudden's Complete Guide to Pain-Free Living
by Bonnie Prudden
(New York: Ballantine Books, 1984)

Pain Erasure the Bonnie Prudden Way
by Bonnie Prudden
(New York: M. Evans, 1977)

RESOURCES

Bonnie Prudden, Inc.
P.O. Box 59
Stockbridge, MA 01262
(800) 221-4634
(413) 298-3066
❑ information
❑ referrals
❑ publications
❑ training and certification

Naturopathic Medicine

What Is Naturopathy or Naturopathic Medicine?

Naturopathy, or naturopathic medicine, is a compilation of a wide variety of natural therapeutics and healing techniques. A mixture of traditional folk wisdom and modern science, with its own time-tested therapeutics, naturopathy is based on a belief in *vis medicatrix naturae* or "the healing power of nature." Sometimes licensed as "drugless therapy," its techniques use the curative abilities of nature's elements, such as sun, water, air, and earth. Many naturopathic physicians use modern medical methods, such as laboratory tests and X rays, too.

In naturopathic medicine, symptoms are viewed as signs that the body is attempting to heal itself. Treatment addresses the underlying cause of illness, primarily unfavorable habits of lifestyle. The individual is treated as an integrated whole. In states where it is legal, naturopathic medicine is a primary care medicine. Scope of practice can range from obstetrics to geriatrics, depending on the expertise of the naturopathic physician.

History and Development of Naturopathy

Nature-based treatment dates back to the dawn of healing, when people first began formally to use the elements and forces of nature to cure. Herbal remedies, therapeutic diets, hydrotherapy (water cures), exercise, and other natural techniques were passed down from the Egyptians to the Greeks. Hippocrates believed in working in harmony with the natural laws that govern homeostasis, the body's drive to return to a state of equilibrium in health.

The term naturopathy was coined by a nineteenth-century

German homeopath, John H. Scheel, to connote health promotion and treatment of the whole person with natural means. Naturopathy emerged as a separate profession when a committee of Kneipp practitioners met in 1900 and decided to broaden their practices to include all available natural methods of healing.

These therapists were followers of Sebastian Kneipp, one of many contributors to the nineteenth-century nature cure movement. Father Kneipp had developed a system of hydrotherapy in Europe in the late 1800s. His techniques included walking barefoot on wet grass early in the morning and running on freshly fallen snow, followed by receiving a brisk dry massage to increase circulation. Besides water cures, his system included therapies based on light, fresh air, and herbal teas.

Today in Germany, the nature cure movement and herbal remedies tradition have matured into a well-established health care practice, with about 5,000 professionals throughout the country. Herr Karl-Heinz Kreussel has built his private practice in Braunsweig to equal that of any modern doctor's. He belongs to one of the regional professional organizations and has published articles in that group's magazine. As a Health Practitioner *(Heilpraktiker)* sanctioned by law, he can use any unregulated materials as part of his treatments. Kreussel, who trained under both an herbalist and an M.D., uses iridology, standard laboratory tests, and clinical examinations to determine his course of treatment.

One Kneipp practitioner, Benedict Lust, emigrated to America to begin teaching and practicing naturopathy here. By 1902, he had founded The American School of Naturopathy in New York City. The practice quickly spread across the United States; California was the first state to pass a law regulating natural medicine, in 1909.

Numerous schools offering a variety of trainings cropped up and disappeared. The movement peaked in America around 1950 and nearly died out by the early 1960s. The legal climate for naturopathy turned cold in many states, in the face of the powerful modern medical establishment. While naturopathic medicine is now legal in six states and the District of Columbia, many naturopaths practicing in other states are old-timers, practicing under their original "Drugless Therapy" licenses, issued before laws prohibiting new naturopathic practices went into effect.

Today, there are only two schools of naturopathic medicine

in the United States: the American College in Portland, Oregon, and John Bastyr College in Seattle, Washington. The American Association of Naturopathic Physicians is beginning to organize and unify the profession, with its own definition and philosophy of modern naturopathic medicine. Alaska, Arizona, Connecticut, Oregon, Washington, and Hawaii recognize naturopathy as a primary medicine with specific licensing laws, as do the Canadian provinces of British Columbia, Manitoba, Ontario, and Saskatchewan. In several other states, efforts are underway to gain licensure for naturopaths.

How Does Naturopathy Work?

Naturopathy's aim is to induce health by making the individual more resilient, the immune system stronger. The first step is to prevent, or intervene in, the development of disease through a variety of natural health care methods.

Three basic principles of naturopathy state that:

❏ The body has a natural drive to maintain equilibrium; symptoms are indications that the body is striving to heal itself and return to that equilibrium.

❏ The root of all disease is the accumulation of waste products, toxins, and bodily refuse due to poor lifestyle habits.

❏ The body contains the wisdom and the power to heal itself, provided that we what we do enhances rather than interferes with this power.

Naturopathic medicine is the West's version of the many other nature-based and holistic medical systems in the world. Like Ayurveda, Traditional Chinese Medicine, and other natural health systems, naturopathy often relies heavily on diet management and herbal remedies. Each shares similar beliefs in promoting health through the regulation of what we eat and drink and of our lifestyles, and uses diet and exercise therapeutically. Like Ayurvedic medicine, naturopathy uses fasting, massage, and enemas or colonics to aid the body in cleansing itself.

Naturopaths often view themselves as teachers more than

doctors, educating their patients in ways to support the body's task of healing itself. The naturopathic physician may counsel clients on the parts of their lifestyles that are depleting their bodies' innate health. For general health maintenance, the naturopath can get you started on the road to better lifestyle practices.

Many people adopt natural health promotion practices on their own as part of self-help programs. There are hundreds of books covering a wide range of natural therapeutics, from herbal remedies and massage to water cures and yoga. Then, for more serious health questions, people turn to the naturopathic doctor.

Naturopathic training includes the study of anatomy, physiology, microbiology, clinical diagnosis, biochemistry, pathology, immunology, pharmacology, gynecology, pediatrics, radiology, cardiology, orthopedics, gastroenterology, minor surgery, and clinical nutrition, and involves taking nearly twice as many hours of psychology as in the typical modern medical school in America.

In addition, naturopaths study a core of natural therapeutics, including homeopathy, botanical medicine (herbals), Chinese medicine, hydrotherapy, and naturopathic manipulative therapy. The scope of therapeutic techniques can vary, depending on the training experience and orientation of the naturopathic physician.

Natural medicine seems to be free of any rigid or built-in orthodoxy. There are no objections in the naturopathic community to teaming with other healing techniques, as is done at the prominent British institution, the School of Naturopathy and Osteopathy. Some naturopaths practice soft-tissue and osseous manipulation or acupuncture in addition to naturopathy. In states that do not license naturopathy or prohibit its practice, they get licensed in a certified medical practice and combine it with their natural therapies in their approach with clients.

Ask the naturopath about his trainings and certifications and what he considers his areas of expertise. The therapeutics a naturopath offers depends on his training, but includes (though is not necessarily limited to):

❏ Physiotherapy: using light, water, ultrasound, electricity, heat, and cold

❏ Therapeutic exercise: yoga or breathing techniques

❏ Chiropractic or osteopathic manipulation of joints and soft tissues, and spinal manipulation

❏ Reflexology, acupressure, or massage

❏ Minor surgery

❏ Acupuncture

❏ Hydrotherapies

❏ Biofeedback, meditation, or autogenic training

❏ Corrective nutrition

❏ Herbal remedies

❏ Supplements, such as vitamins, minerals, glandular extracts, hormones, and enzymes

❏ Homeopathic remedies

What Happens in a Session?

As with most medical systems, the first session begins with the naturopath taking the patient's history and making a clinical diagnosis. Naturopaths spend an extensive amount of time doing this to help them understand both the physical and psychological roots of the patient's current health disorder(s). The naturopathic physician may order lab tests, and even an X ray or ultrasound, if necessary. Many will perform an osteopathic diagnosis, checking for misaligned structure or posture, or tender spots. One of the most important consultations concerns the patient's diet. The client may fill out a three- or five-day record of food intake for nutrient analysis.

Then the patient and doctor discuss options for treatment and set up a program. The physician often emphasizes psychological health and stress reduction because of their positive effects on the body. The purpose is to intervene in the disease process and/or help the patient reorganize his lifestyle to support an innate healing process. Depending on the severity of the condition, the healing program may be a mixture of home remedies, such as herbal teas and hot baths, homeopathic remedies, and office visits, for acupuncture, colonics, massages, osteopathic manipulations, or other treatment specialties.

Applications and Cautions

Naturopathy can be used to treat almost all but the most acute diseases. Natural therapeutics can help heal such disorders as sore throats and the common cold, flu, colitis, gastritis, bronchitis, piles, and digestive and liver problems. Naturopathy has also aided some serious conditions, such as tuberculosis.

Treatment is often dictated by the patient's willingness to change or participate. If you are reluctant or unwilling to work as a partner with your naturopath and follow the program the two of you devise, the benefits of naturopathy may be limited.

As primary care providers, naturopathic physicians also know to refer a patient to a specialist when the disease is out of their areas of expertise or better served by modern medicine. Health crises, such as acute and massive infections, appendicitis, broken limbs, and gaping wounds are the domain of allopathic medicine's swift and interventive techniques.

READ MORE ABOUT IT

NATUROPATHIC MEDICINE

Traditional Foods are Your Best Medicine: Health and Longevity with the Animal, Sea and Vegetable Foods of Our Ancestors
by Ronald F. Schmid, N.D.
(Stratford, CT: Ocean View Publications, 1987)

Everywoman's Book
by Paava Airola, N.D., Ph.D.
(Phoenix, AZ: Health Plus Publishers, 1979)

RESOURCES

American Association of Naturopathic Physicians
P.O. Box 2579
Kirkland, WA 98083-2579
(206) 827-6035
❏ state association list
❏ publications
❏ conference

National College of Naturopathic Medicine
11231 S.E. Market Street
Portland, OR 97216
(503) 255-4860
❏ information
❏ training and certification
❏ clinic
❏ CEU seminars
❏ presentations
❏ research

John Bastyr College
144 N.E. 54th Street
Seattle, WA 98105
(206) 523-9585
❏ information
❏ training and certification

Nutrition and Nutrition Therapies

What Are Nutrition and Nutrition Therapies?

Nutrition is the process of supplying or receiving nourishment. It is the food we put, or do not put, in our mouths to feed the body—and the mind and soul, as well.

People's habits about food today range from a heavy consumption of highly processed or fast foods with questionable nutritional value to a multitude of healthier regimens, such as vegetarianism and organic health food diets. Both ends of the nutrition continuum have growing food industries.

Beyond general nourishment, food and diet have been used throughout history as effective tools in preventive and therapeutic medicine. Recently we have begun to recognize once again and to investigate the valuable role that nutrition can play in a comprehensive health program. Nutrition therapies, such as Orthomolecular Medicine/Psychiatry, are used to help treat diseases like schizophrenia. Bookstores are bursting with choices for both weight-reduction and disease-prevention diets.

And beyond the commercialism, competition, and controversies surrounding nutrition theories, there is a growing awareness of eating disorders. Some counselors are helping clients examine their eating habits, the way these individuals relate to food, and the psychoemotional issues underlying nourishment and food abuse.

It would take at least an entire book to survey and explain the development and workings of the many approaches to nutrition and nutrition therapies. This chapter is an overview of this burgeoning field, highlighting only a few of the overwhelming number of choices.

History and Development of Nutrition and Food Therapies

In primitive times, obtaining and eating food consumed most of humanity's time and energy. Food is so basic to life that, along with herbs, it was our first medicine. Garlic was a cure for many maladies in Egypt, Babylonia, Greece, and other cradles of civilization. The ancients prescribed it for respiratory infections, intestinal disorders, wounds, insect bites, and skin disorders.

Cabbage is a folk medicine remedy for headaches, colic, and ulcers. Hippocrates recommended cooked cabbage for heart and bowel disease. In France in the 1800s, several incidents were recorded of crushed and gangrenous legs that were saved from amputation by wrapping the wounds with cabbage leaves.

In the 1700s, every English ship began carrying lime or lemon juice to prevent and treat scurvy, an affliction of sailors long at sea. That is how the British sailor got the nickname "limey." Two hundred years later, scientists discovered the substances in citrus fruit that prevented scurvy and other diseases—by studying rice. Christian Eijkman, a Dutch medical officer in the East Indies, examined people in prison camps. He showed that prisoners who ate polished rice got beriberi. People who ate whole rice, hull and all, did not. A Polish biochemist in London, Casimir Funk, isolated the anti-beriberi factor contained in rice hulls, a factor also contained in citrus fruit, that he thought belonged to a class of chemicals called *amines*. He coined the term *vitamine*, meaning "amine essential to life."

By the early 1900s, the scientific community had dropped the *e* on Funk's term and discovered an alphabet soup of separate vitamins. Dr. Albert Szent-Gyorgi of Hungary and Dr. Charles King of Pittsburgh were the first to isolate vitamin C in lemons. A University of Wisconsin biochemist, E. V. McCollum, discovered the first fat-soluble vitamin, vitamin A.

Earlier, back in the 1820s, an army surgeon had been trying to figure out what happened to food once we swallowed it. William Beaumont was fortunate enough to treat a soldier for a gunshot wound that did not heal completely, leaving a permanent hole in his side—and stomach. Beaumont kept the poor man under observation for ten years, peering into his stomach to study its lining and the flow of gastric juices. He would dip pieces of meat and other foods through the stomach fistula to see how long it would take to digest them. The experiments made a big contribution to metabolic and digestive research, if not to that soldier's well-being. (Finally the man left Beaumont, went to Canada, married and raised a family. Beaumont had to hire him back and negotiate better working conditions to do follow-up studies some years later.)

Metabolic researchers were putting together a picture of proteins, carbohydrates, and fats, as well as vitamins and minerals, as essential to human life and health. By the 1940s, scientists had identified more than 40 nutrients contained in foods, including 13 vitamins. They also determined that we need minerals, such as calcium, iron and potassium, to regulate various body functions. The wartime food-enrichment program gave a boost to an already growing tendency to advertise the vitamin power of food products. Even chocolate bars were hyped for their nutrient value!

The '50s and early '60s was the era of fortified cereals on the one hand and the beginning of what was called "food faddism" on the other. While Wonder Bread built our bodies 12 ways, nutritionists like Adele Davis were trying to put their fingers—and books—into the dike in a fight against the rising flood of processed foods. How many kids had to suffer through Tiger's Milk (skim milk with orange juice and brewer's yeast) for breakfast?

The cultural convulsion of the '60s inspired some people to dump airy white bread for nuts and fruit. While some abused their bodies with drugs, others in this generation sparked a back-to-nature movement. These baby boomers now fuel the health movement. Whether its a light meal of salad or sushi after an aerobics class or a taste of spa cuisine at a health resort, eating healthy is in. Besides turning Woodstockers into Live-Aid hunger relief fund-raisers, baby boomers have turned health foods into a sophisticated natural foods industry, supporting the growing organic food and megavitamins markets.

In 1968, Stanford chemistry professor Linus Pauling published a paper in the prestigious journal *Science*. He discussed creating an optimum molecular environment in the mind by providing the right concentration of specific biochemicals such as vitamins. He coined the term *orthomolecular* to mean optimum, or right (ortho), molecules.

Nontraditional scientists adopted Pauling's principles, applying them first to mental disorders and then to physical illness and general health. The controversial fields of Orthomolecular Psychiatry and Orthomolecular Medicine were created. Doctors treated patients with special diets and supplements which were individualized, depending on the client's problems and needs. While dieticians and conventional medical doctors were still talking about the basic food groups, orthomolecular nutritionists were prescribing huge doses of vitamins. Doctors used biochemicals to correct nutritional deficiencies they saw as factors in many physical and mental diseases.

Evidence for nutrient factors in mental disease was not new. As early as 1952, Doctors Abram Hoffer and Humphreys Osmond observed that schizophrenics improved greatly when given 17 grams (1,000 times the recommended daily allowance) of niacin or niacinamide. Hoffer suggested that there were two types of vitamin shortages in humans. In the first type, the staple diet does not provide enough of the nutrient. This causes vitamin deficiencies that may lead to diseases, such as scurvy (lack of vitamin C) and pellagra (lack of niacin). In the second type, the body is unable to absorb or otherwise metabolize adequate doses of vitamins from the foods eaten, resulting in a deficiency that may underline some physical and mental health problems.

Both the American Psychiatry Association and the Alberta (Canada) College of Physicians looked into the megavitamin controversy and found little convincing evidence for the new orthomolecular theory. The toxic potential of vitamin A and several incidents of vitamin overdoses are often cited in debates about vitamin therapies. In 1977, the *Canadian Medical Association Journal* called for more clinical studies.

In 1976, a bill sponsored by Senator William Proxmire (D-Wisconsin) curtailed the FDA's regulatory powers over dietary supplements. Now, vitamins can be sold over the counter and labeling requirements are minimal. The Consumer's Union sees this lack of regulation as a marketer's paradise and a consumer's Pandora's box. Though producers still must maintain truth in advertising, CU notes that editorial articles can make all sorts of unsubstantiated or inadequately proven claims about miraculous vitamin cures.

While legislative and scientific battles raged over dietary deficiencies, nutrition ignorance, and appropriate treatment modalities, the battle of the bulge was waged at bookstores and on bathroom scales. The diet craze hit big in the '70s and '80s. Dr. Robert Atkins and Dr. Nathan Pritikin, and even ritzy suburbs like Beverly Hills and Scarsdale, had their own diets. Debate still continues over whether a high carbohydrate/low protein or a high protein/low carbohydrate diet is better. Dr. Nathan Pritikin popularized the notion of Preventative Medicine not only by awakening the dieting public to his "medically sound" eating and exercise routines, but by attracting doctors to his Longevity Center and raising their consciousness about nutrition's role in health maintenance.

Various national associations have published research findings on the benefits of restricting sodium, eating oat bran and fiber, or substituting saturated fats with polyunsaturates. Quick to exploit anything that will motivate sales, commercial food producers have been touting the cancer-, heart disease–, and cholesterol-prevention factors in their products ever since.

In 1982, California passed strict guidelines for the advertising and labeling of agricultural commodities and processed food products that use terms like "organic," "organically grown," and "wild." Legitimate organic growers and health food outlets began participating in a cooperative self-regulation system, policing growing conditions and labeling, and giving consumers assurance that what they are buying is truly organic. When public figures such as Ralph Nader and Meryl Streep stirred up media interest in the cancer-causing potential of pesticides, there were boomlets of media stories on "safe" foods. Now, produce testing for pesticide residue for a number of major grocery store chains has developed into a growing cottage industry.

Traditional diet programs and self-help groups continue to give weight watchers and overeaters the social and emotional support needed to change their eating habits, if not their lives. Some residential treatment centers offer help for people with eating disorders. More information on the effects of nutrients and the role food plays in a person's life is available. The wider range of food options and nutritional philosophies and therapies underscores the point that food can indeed be some of the best medicine.

Nutrition Therapies and Food Philosophies

There are many dietary practices and lifestyle suggestions from which to choose once the decision has been made to focus on eating habits and nutrition. The consumer must wade through mounds of information—and aggressive advertising—to distinguish between food faddism and appropriate food technology. A growing number of health professionals offer various nutrition therapies. There are also many options for preventative nutrition programs. And increasingly, people are looking at the role food and nourishment play in their emotional lives.

That old saying, "What is one man's meat is another's poison," is as true today as it was 2,000 years ago when the Roman philosopher Lucretius wrote it in his epic poem *On the Nature of Things*. People not only have different tastes in food, they also have a variety of metabolisms that deal with nutrients at different rates and in different ways.

Nobel laureate Pauling has proposed a range for Recommended Daily Intake, to allow for individual variability in nutrient needs. Testifying before a Senate subcommittee on health, he suggested that the Recommended Dietary Allowances of vitamins and minerals set by the Food and Nutrition Board of the FDA was misleading. He argued that the term should be MDA, for Minimum Dietary Allowance because, he said, the current RDA levels were closer to the amount that merely prevents death or serious vitamin deficiency diseases, as opposed to the higher amount that will actually help maintain optimum health.

Pauling was echoing the findings of University of Texas biochemist Roger Williams, discoverer of pantothenic and folic acids, both part of the B-complex vitamin group. Williams is the proponent of "biochemical individuality," the idea that everybody has different nutrient requirements to avoid disease and achieve optimum health. He listed 40 "growth and maintenance chemicals" in his 1977 classic work *The Wonderful World Within You: Your Inner Nutritional Environment*. These nutrients are not only key to preventative nutrition, they are also the ammunition that doctors use to combat diseases in therapeutic nutrition.

Doctors practicing Orthomolecular Medicine and its cousin, Clinical Ecology, look at a patient's nutrient deficiencies and imbalances. Orthomolecular physicians adjust concentrations of "right molecules," of such vital nutrients as vitamins, minerals, trace elements, amino acids, enzymes, and hormones, to treat underlying factors in infectious and degenerative diseases. Their focus is on the microenvironment of cells. Optimal nutrient balance promotes proper functioning of the body's internal systems, which are normally geared to handle most disease conditions.

Clinical ecologists incorporate everything from cellular science to environmental ecology in their theories. They focus on all maladaptive reactions—mental, physical, emotional, social—that are a result of exposure to food, chemicals, and other pollutants. In his book, *Brain Allergies*, orthomolecular psychiatrist William Philpott explains how Clinical Ecology deals with patients with acute localized effects (e.g., asthma, eczema, gastrointestinal allergies), acute systemic effects (e.g., headaches, fatigue, neuralgia), and acute mental effects (e.g., confusion, depression, hallucinations).

Physicians practicing what he calls a "toximolecular" approach to medicine use a battery of lab tests to help make their diagnoses. These tests measure things like sugar tolerance, thyroid function, blood levels of vitamins and minerals, insulin levels, and other conditions. They may use hair analysis to evaluate body levels of trace minerals and look at dietary habits, often analyzing a three- to five-day food intake for nutrients and calories. Some doctors counsel patients to clean house and give up certain foods to avoid allergens (reaction-causing agents). Others choose to take the offensive, using nutrient megadoses and other therapies, such as rotation eating, to build up the patient's immune system and general health.

People looking for a sensible eating plan to avoid crisis conditions, such as food allergies, have a wide range of philosophies and diets to explore. The health movement accommodates diverse outlooks. We have heard of everything from *Life Extension* (popular with the muscle-building crowd) and *Fit for Life* (which integrates the ideas of food combining and body cycles) to fasting and the spiritual, ecological, and metabolic benefits of vegetarianism.

The rising popularity of Eastern traditions has also brought a new consciousness about the powers of food beyond the physical. Many people have adopted and adapted nutritional traditions from India, China, and Japan. Not only do these systems talk about balancing the energies of food, described in each indigenous system's language, but they promote eating as part of an overall attitude and approach to life and health. Ayurveda, for example, sees food as an integral part of preventive health practices, therapeutic treatment, spiritual balance, and optimum mental functioning.

The Oriental systems organize food—its energies, flavors and actions—by the principle of yin/yang and elements. George Ohsawa invented Macrobiotics from the nutritional routine he used to cure his tuberculosis. Macrobiotic food philosophy centers on grains, especially brown rice, believing they act as balancing energies between yin foods (e.g., sugars and fruit) and yang foods (e.g., meat).

Western approaches to balancing food include food combining and acid-alkaline awareness. Food combining takes into account the various lengths of time and competing enzymes required for the digestive system to process different types of food. Vegetables can be consumed with proteins. Those enzymes work together. Meat and potatoes, however, is not an efficient combination. In fact, the reason this classic American meal "sticks to the ribs" is because the digestive system will leave most meats putrefying in the stomach for an hour or two while it processes the starches first, especially if the potato was swimming in butter.

Eating too many acid-producing foods (like meat, dairy products, and grains) produces mucus, which clogs the system. Stuffy noses, sluggish intestines, decreased oxygenation in the bloodstream, and diminished mental clarity might signal too many acid-forming foods in the diet. An increased consumption of alkaline-based foods can counteract these effects. Proponents of this pH balancing approach to food are big on vegetables, especially the leafy green ones.

Most food philosophies and diets warn about the consequences of overeating. Dietary excess leads to digestive overload. When the body is given either too much of a specific substance or simply a general onslaught of food, the digestive organs must work overtime. With too much work, the system goes into stress. Everything slows down.

Extra carbohydrates ferment and form gas. Proteins putrefy, releasing uric acid. These toxic byproducts upset the intestinal ecosystem, creating flatulence, constipation, and other signs of eliminative imbalance. Undigested fat particles become rancid and collect as cholesterol. General physiological functioning is impeded. A clogged colon blocks the body's efficient cleansing system. Metabolic waste products collect, creating edema in body tissues, making the body look and feel puffy. A general feeling of malaise can pervade body and mind. That, in turn, can trigger a whole new cycle of food abuse.

Food philosophies also consider food's effect on the mind. Reactions can range from the physical to the emotional. Most people have at some point experienced "sugar highs" and "sugar blues," and understand implicitly the effects that too many sweets can have on one's mood, energy, and physical functioning.

Spiritual aspirants avoid certain foods believed to interfere with energy balance and meditation practice. For instance, followers of Ayurveda see onions as too stimulating. On the other hand, most other vegetables and fruits are inherently balanced and harmonious, conducive to clear thinking and meditation.

Many food philosophies acknowledge that we elevate food to a high level of importance in our lives. Specific foods have religious significance. Wine and bread are ritually consumed by Christians during Communion. Jews keep kosher, Hindus do not eat beef, and Moslems and Jews avoid pork. Food also symbolizes mother's love, good times with good friends, and socioeconomic status. Real men don't eat quiche and the rich can afford caviar.

People involved in the holistic health movement learn to shift their perspectives on food. While they clean up their acts on a calorie and nutrient level, they also learn to acknowledge how their eating habits symbolize their approaches to nourishment in general. Nourishment is seen as more than just the process of providing nutrients to the body. It is also emotional and spiritual. Food expresses one's experience of or approach to nurturance— the ability to feed and grow, cherish and promote, love and sustain oneself.

Alternately, individuals with severe psychological or physical problems misuse food in highly self-destructive ways. Anorexics obsess over imagined fat and deny themselves nourishment. Bulimics stuff down feelings with food and then throw it all back up. Obese overeaters nibble or gorge, trying to fill a void, and can't get enough. Whether emotionally or chemically triggered, physical cravings for favorite treats drive people to abuse food. The abuse further stresses the body and disturbs the mind.

Clinical ecologists, eating disorder specialists, and various holistically-oriented therapists have been working with clients whose weight problems and allergies turn out to be a tip of an iceberg of psychoemotional and biochemical imbalances. These people have real, physically-based disorders that expose significant messages about their lives.

Ultimately, whether pushed into awareness and action by the crisis of physical illness, by weight problems, by an eating disorder, or by age, nutrition awareness is an issue almost everyone will face at some time in his or her life. We are sometimes hostages of marketeers, and often at the mercy of social obligations and habits. Getting clear about what are good or optimal habits can be a complex process.

The first step is to recognize all the various diets, philosophies, and therapies as tools for reaching a health goal. The next step is to get support for the process of changing personal tastes, habits, and emotional perspectives on food and nurturance. Support can involve getting information and counseling, or just having good friends to talk with when under stress.

My experience with food, weight concerns, allergies, cooking, and nurturance issues has led me to believe that "diets" can cause a lot of problems. Food philosophies are complex, tough to understand and follow in the beginning—and they require commitment and an investment of time and energy. Nutrition therapies often are no less complicated, and they tend to be followed more devotedly when they are used as part of the treatment for some medical condition. There is nothing like fear to fuel motivation.

I found that support groups, therapy, and/or a journal give the kind of outside perspective needed in sorting out eating habits. For me, a nutrition psychologist would have made things a lot easier—someone, that is, who understands the entanglements of food, nurturance, love, rewards, personality, family dynamics, and nutrients. Then again, I might have opted for six months at a good health spa too, if I could have afforded it. Those places do all the cooking and keep you busy with exercise, massage, and play. And they know how to make healthy food look and taste interesting, if not as good as the ice cream, bagels, and chocolate you left behind.

Ultimately, you have to find an approach that not only fits your budget, but your specific needs, lifestyle, and level of commitment as well. A sudden, cold turkey change in diet and eating habits may be effective for some stalwart types, but for others it can be overwhelming to the point of uselessness. A well-considered and methodical approach, backed by support wherever you can get it, is often the best way to implement a nutritional program that is both nourishing and nurturing.

READ MORE ABOUT IT

NUTRITION AND NUTRITION THERAPIES

Orthomolecular Nutrition: New Lifestyles for Super Good Health
by Abram Hoffer, Ph.D., M.D. and Morton Walker, D.P.M.
(New Canaan, CT: Keats Publishing, 1978)

Brain Allergies: The Psychonutrient Connection
by William H. Philpott, M.D. and Dwight K. Kalita, Ph.D.
(New Canaan, CT: Keats Publishing, 1980)

Food Power
by George Schwartz, M.D.
(New York: McGraw Hill, 1979)

Natural Healing Through Macrobiotics
by Michio Kushi
(Tokyo: Japan Publications, 1979)

Food is Your Best Medicine
by Henry G. Bieler, M.D.
(New York: Random House, 1966)

Chinese System of Food Cures: Prevention and Remedies
by Henry C. Lu
(New York: Sterling Publishing, 1986)

An Alternative Approach to Allergies
by Theron G. Randolph, M.D. and Ralph W. Moss, Ph.D.
(New York: Lippincott & Crowell, 1979)

Spiritual Nutrition and the Rainbow Diet
by Gabriel Cousens, M.D.
(Boulder, CO: Cassandra Press, 1986)

The Wonderful World Within You: Your Inner Nutritional Environment
by Dr. Roger Williams
(New York: Bantam Books, 1977)

The Eating Gorilla Comes in Peace: The Transcendental Principles of Life Applied to Diet and the Regenerative Discipline of True Health
by Bubba Free John
(Middletown, CA: The Dawn Horse Press, 1979)

Fit for Life
by Harvey and Marilyn Diamond
(New York: Warner Books, 1985)

Life Extension: A Practical Scientific Approach
by Durk Pearson and Sandy Shaw
(New York: Warner Books, 1982)

Detox
by Phyllis Saifer, M.D., M.P.H. and Merla Zellerbach
(Los Angeles: Jeremy P. Tarcher, 1984)

RESOURCES

North American Vegetarian Society
P.O. Box 72
Dodgerville, NY 13329
(518) 568-7970
❏ information
❏ local organization referral
❏ publications
❏ membership

Kushi Institute (macrobiotics)
17 Station Street
Brookline Village, MA 02147
(617) 738-0045
❏ information
❏ classes

Past Life Therapy

What Is Past Life or Regression Therapy?

Past Life Therapy (PLT) is the accessing of information or images from possible former lifetimes, usually through hypnotic regression or some form of altered state of consciousness, for therapeutic purposes. Past Life *Therapy* differs from Past Life *Regression* in the use and meaning of the past life information.

Past life regression is a general term for probing the unconscious mind to retrieve *historical* memories or information, from childhood or previous lives. The late Helen Wambaugh conducted thousands of past life regressions to collect historical data—past and *future*—to investigate the theory of reincarnation. Her group regression events were for research and personal experience, not therapy. Subjects had no expectation of follow-up counseling to help them understand and deal with the information.

Past life therapy searches emotionally or physically traumatic life memories for therapeutic purposes, such as promoting cathartic release, reframing attitudes, changing old habits or behavior problems, and gaining conscious insight into the lessons of that life or memory. Therapists use past life regression as *one of* the therapeutic tools or techniques available to them to help clients resolve their problems. These therapists may call their practices Regression Therapy or Transformational Therapy.

History and Development of Past Life Therapy

The psychotherapeutic use of past lives arose during this century out of a confluence of two diverse traditions meeting in the West. A truly transpersonal psychology ("beyond the per-

227

sona or mask"), Past Life Therapy developed from a growing awareness of ancient spiritual traditions and experimental psychologies.

The concept of past lives or reincarnation has been around since the beginning of human culture, recorded in pictures, words, and cryptic symbols by peoples ranging from the Egyptians and Tibetans to Christian Gnostics and Native Americans. Reincarnation is the belief in the survival of the soul beyond the life of the body. The Egyptians mummified bodies and buried servants with their rulers so their afterlives would be as rich as their earthbound lives. The Hindus believe we live cycles of birth and death, including lives as animals before reincarnation as humans, progressing up an evolutionary path.

The early pioneers in past life therapy came from several different fields and philosophical roots. Colonel Albert de Roches, who claimed to have regressed patients back beyond childhood to *in utero* and previous life memories, was a turn-of-the-century French psychoanalyst and hypnotherapist. Edgar Cayce, the American clairvoyant venerated as "the sleeping prophet" because he gave medical readings and other advice while in a trance, was simple country folk. His channeling often connected past lives to present health problems, though his limited education and strict religious upbringing rejected many of the concepts he communicated while channeling.

While the '50s saw the public entertained with regression stories, such as the case of Bridey Murphy, and a debate on proof of reincarnation, past life therapy was quietly taking shape. An English psychiatrist, Dr. Denys Kelsey, began exploring reincarnation as an explanation for behavior problems when more conventional therapeutic approaches had failed. A member of the Royal College of Physicians, Kelsey was one of the first to go public with his use of prenatal and past life regressions.

Morris Netherton, whom many consider one of the founders of Past Life Therapy, documented past life traumas affecting current life health conditions. His 1978 book, *Past Life Therapy,* relates case studies of chronic illnesses such as migraines, ulcers, and epilepsy.

However, in the '70s, the American public really took note of the philosophical underpinnings of past lives with Dr. Raymond Moody's ground-breaking study of Near Death Experiences (NDEs) in *Life After Life*. While several other explanations for NDEs are proposed and may be possible, Moody's work, and further research by Kenneth Ring, Ph.D., have opened wider the window to belief in survival of the soul.

Meanwhile, the field of psychotherapy was beginning to shift from the cognitive and interpretive "talk therapy" to more experimental forms. These theoretical developments validated what past life therapists were finding themselves. Hypnotherapists, for example, had discovered the use of spontaneous images of other lives to release emotional and physical traumas to help clients overcome mental and physical health problems.

Hazel Denning, Ph.D., one of the founders of the Association for Past-Life Research and Therapy (APRT), is a quintessential example of the kind of regression therapist coming to the fore. Her first regression into a past life was an accident. A client's hypnotic regression to childhood overshot and spontaneously landed in a life during the Civil War. Like most hypnotherapists who have experienced a similar surprise, Denning recovered enough to use the imagery therapeutically with her client, achieving positive results. Typically, she did not talk about it for a long time but used the technique with success on other clients.

Denning is now executive director of APRT, an organization established in 1980 for past life therapists to come together and share experiences, research, and expertise. APRT holds an annual conference for professionals and knowledgeable laypersons, publishes the *Journal of Regression Therapy,* and trains clinicians interested in incorporating past life therapeutic techniques into their practices.

Two of APRT's members are leaders in a developing branch of PLT, Clinical Depossession. William Baldwin, Ph.D. and Edith Fiore, Ph.D. have presented fascinating stories of single-entity and multiple-entity possessions. These are cases where wandering souls take up residency in a living person—sometimes more than one soul in a single person! Possessions in these cases are not quite so dramatic as the pea soup–spitting and head-spinning demon in the movie *The Exorcist.* However, disembodied souls that don't know how (or refuse) to leave earth and go into the light can contribute to or cause emotional, behavioral, and health problems.

How Regression Therapy Works

Whether the past lives are real or metaphorical stories, PLT is based on the concept of reincarnation or survival of the soul, and that the images relate to traumas that can be resolved. One does not necessarily need to believe in the philosophy to benefit from regression material. The information can be used to resolve deeply buried attitudes, beliefs, or experiences affecting current life problems.

Stanislav Grof, a leading researcher in experiential psychology, is particularly known for his theoretical work on the influence of the birth experience on personality and health. He has found that we humans carry major unconscious imprints of physical accidents and emotional traumas, including the birth experience.

In therapy, these imprints are called complexes. Complexes are psychic, emotional, and physical impressions laid down as life is lived. The new psychologies recognize that we "embody" our complexes—express them through many parts of ourselves. Traumatic influences can show up as a physical symptom, a neurotic complaint or behavior, a dream, or even a secondary personality.

PLT extends these concepts to past lives. Jungian psychotherapist Roger Woolger marries the idea of Grof's imprints with complexes and extends both back before conception. In his 1987 book, *Other Lives, Other Selves,* he proposes that psychic content can be inherited, not just through the genes but also through some other energetic level, from previous lives. Woolger believes he has treated "past life complexes" as well as current life ones in his practice.

The mechanism for transmitting these imprints or impressions is not certain. Theories abound. So do proposals for what else these past life memories may be:

❏ Daydreaming or fantasizing: we do it all the time.

❏ Cryptomnesia: forgetting that you read or heard it and remembering the information as your own memory.

❏ Fraud: conscious or unconscious story-telling for recognition or other kinds of reward.

❏ Collective unconscious: tapping into Jung's concept of the universal group memory or images, but seeing them as your own.

❏ Inherited memory: imaging memories (genetic or cellular) of a lineal descendent or a related personality.

❏ Clairvoyance and telepathy: picking up images or knowledge from other living people and reading it as your own memory.

❏ Mediumistic possession: projected images of a deceased person who has taken over your mind.

Real or metaphysical, the material clients bring into the session can give insight to personality, behavior problems, deeply buried memories and emotions, attitudes and beliefs about themselves and their lives. Further, people undergoing past life therapy focus on using these insights to change themselves, their attitudes, and their lives. The added philosophical bonus is that if they believe in reincarnation, the work they do on themselves in this life is part of moving further along their particular evolutionary or spiritual path. Psychological healing is part of spiritual growth.

What Happens in a Past Life Therapy Session?

Actual regression starts with induction into an altered state. This can be either a light state, such as when doing visual imagery, or a deeper state, often identified with hypnosis (see Hypnosis). The therapist will guide you back through childhood, birth, and womb time to a life that relates to whatever issue you have agreed to explore. When you have arrived at a time and place, the regressor will probably ask you to describe what you see, your surroundings and other people, your own body and what you are feeling. This helps anchor the images or impressions and bring them into focus.

What actually transpires after that is as varied as the style of the therapist and the images and experience the client is relating. Several points to remember:

❏ The therapist is watching over you and your experience, creating a safe environment for you to explore deep images and emotions.

❑ You can come out of the altered state whenever you choose to.

❑ You may see images, hear sounds or voices, smell odors, or just get thoughts; each of us has our own way of seeing and knowing.

❑ You should keep up communication with the regressor so she can guide you and help you if the experience is confusing or scary.

❑ You do not necessarily have to dramatize or act out what you are experiencing, but letting out the tears, laughter, or anger may be very therapeutic. Let your therapist be your guide.

All of the APRT therapists I worked with, in a year-long experiment and in subsequent sessions, directed me each time to look at three important points in the lives examined:

❑ Just before death: describing the circumstances and reasons.

❑ Just before dying: my dying thoughts, emotions and decisions made in that transitional moment.

❑ Just after the moment of death: rising above the drama of the life and death to look at what I might learn by my actions or by acting and feeling differently.

These three insights usually captured the meaning of each life and death. I saw emotional decisions, judgments I made about being a man or a woman, feelings of hate, anger, or guilt, and assumptions about life that were locked in at the moment of death. I also understood what I could learn from these scenes by taking a different attitude or giving up those reactive decisions. The lessons almost always related exactly to what I needed to see about a current life problem.

Applications and Cautions

Past life therapy is often reserved for when traditional methods fail to resolve any kind of neurotic complaint through exploration of childhood history. It can also be a catalyst to break through a particular block in dealing with something of either an emotional or physical nature.

Past life therapy's use of imagery and emphasis on and embodiment of our complexes gives it potential for dealing with chronic mental and physical health problems. Its experimental focus for insight and cathartic release helps remove possible sources of emotional, behavioral, and psychosomatic symptoms. Examples of problems that respond particularly well to past life regression therapy include:

❑ Difficulties in relationships: understanding possible reasons for distrust, hurt, anger, and other underlying emotions; when pervasive in a relationship, they block healthy communication stemming from former, past life relationships and incidents.

❑ Trait guilt: chronic guilt, a common emotional reaction to the loss, for example, of loved ones in one or more past lives, carried over to pervade this life's relationships.

❑ Phobias and compulsions: fearful reaction to cigarette smoke, for example, may recall a death by fire; a drive to repeatedly wash your hands may be symbolic of washing off blood from a previous life murder.

❑ Asthma: various past life therapists have found asthma connected to overwhelming pressure from parents as a child, possibly including unexpressed anger, or death by smothering or drowning in a past life.

❑ Chronic back pain: can be a memory or imprint from a stabbing or other violent assault and death, or symbolic of a burden too heavy to carry in a former life.

It is important to point out that these are only examples and usually discovered after medical reasons have been explored and ruled out. And PLT is not for every medical condition, neurotic complaint, or personality.

Some clients might fancy themselves as John Paul Jones or Joan of Arc to avoid looking at possible darker sides of themselves, frustrating the goal of therapy—healing through knowing ourselves. Woolger lists other kinds of clients not well suited for this type of therapy and possible misuses of this therapeutic tool:

❏ The person with schizophrenic tendencies involving a profound denial of present life ("poor reality sense"); PLT would be just another escape.

❏ The person who had a strict religious upbringing where the idea of reincarnation and the other philosophical underpinnings of PLT would offend and distract the client from the therapeutic process.

❏ The person for whom this form of experiential therapy might be too intense or overwhelming; real or metaphorical, exposing such raw emotion might encourage dissociation or the need to defend the conscious mind.

❏ The overintellectual and curious person who might focus on the reality and theories about past lives and not the therapeutic opportunity for facing and healing oneself.

Past life regression and therapy has been a profoundly healing influence in my life. It is also the one tool that has given me the deepest struggles. I know that it is not something to be used lightly.

The most important advice I can give is: make sure you have a deep and trusting relationship with whoever regresses you. This facilitates both deeper, more honest revelations and a safety net in case you need help in coping with the possibly extreme emotions that can surface. The first time I "relived" killing someone (as a barbarian warlord bent on revenge) was scary and shocking. I had nail marks in my hands for hours. I was glad to have the support in accepting that I could feel that angry and violent.

I don't know whether I believe in past lives, whether the many images and stories I have seen for myself are real or products of my very rich and active imagination. I *have* struggled with getting caught up in the drama of these stories at the expense of living my present life in the moment. But most important, I have learned to use the insights gleaned from each session to transform how I feel about myself and other people in my life.

I do believe in some of the core assumptions of past life therapy philosophy as articulated by Denning: There are no good and bad experiences or lives, just opportunities to learn something. Pain is a benevolent signal that something is wrong and needs to be changed. And, I am responsible for my life and the only one who can change and restore its harmony.

Most important, I have learned not to judge other people as they go about learning their lessons. I may avoid the S.O.B. at work, aggressively protect myself from rapists and murderers, and choose not to live the life of a prostitute or monk. However, I do not hate them for their problems and choices; I could have been doing all of the above in other lives!

READ MORE ABOUT IT

PAST LIFE THERAPY

Other Lives, Other Selves: A Jungian Psychotherapist Discovers Past Lives
by Roger J. Woolger, Ph.D.
(New York: Doubleday, 1987)

Reincarnation: A New Horizon in Science, Religion and Society
by Sylvia Cranston and Carey Williams
(New York: Julian Press, 1984)

Reincarnation: The Phoenix Fire Mystery
edited by Joseph Head and S.L. Cranston
(New York: Julian Press/Crown Publishers, 1977)

Past Life Therapy
by Morris Netherton and Nancy Shiffren
(New York: Morrow, 1978)

You Have Been Here Before
by Edith Fiore
(New York: Ballantine, 1979)

RESOURCES

Association for Past-Life Therapies, Inc.
P.O. Box 20151
Riverside, CA 92516
(714) 784-1570
❑ information
❑ conferences
❑ seminars
❑ journal
❑ membership

Polarity
Therapy

What Is Polarity Therapy?

Polarity is a concept based on principles of energy, a bodywork, and a composite healing philosophy based primarily but not exclusively on East Indian Ayurvedic principles. Created by Dr. Randolph Stone, an osteopath, chiropractor, and naturopath, polarity is designed to balance the body's subtle or electromagnetic energy through:

- ❏ touch, working with polarity trigger points
- ❏ stretching exercises, called polarity yoga or polar energetics
- ❏ an approach to eating and nutrition based on the philosophy's principles
- ❏ attitude, mental-emotional balancing

Unlike other bodyworks, Polarity Therapy does not manipulate muscles or bones but works through the body's own energy system by placing hands on the body's energy centers and poles to redirect the flow.

History and Development of Polarity

Dr. Stone was a naturalized American who emigrated to Chicago from Austria as a youth. He spent 50 years studying a diverse range of healing modalities all over the world. Besides certification in chiropractic, osteopathy, and naturopathy, he trained in acupressure, herbology, reflexology, and other Eastern massage techniques. He also gained insight on the subtle electromagnetic fields of the body from studying the work of the sixteenth-century Swiss physician Paracelsus, and settled in India in the late 1950s, where he integrated a lifetime of study, insight, and practice into Polarity Therapy. He wrote several books, traveling back to the U.S. and other parts of the world teaching his new technique and philosophy. Ten years before he died, in 1981, Stone appointed Pierre Pannetier to take over leadership and the future development of the polarity movement. Pannetier traveled the country teaching the polarity techniques until his death in 1984. Several branches of schools of polarity, started by students of Dr. Stone and emphasizing different interpretations of the polarity philosophy, are now uniting under the umbrella of a professional organization, the American Polarity Therapy Association, and creating standards for polarity practices.

How Does Polarity Work?

Polarity seeks to balance the flow of life force through a free-flowing exchange between the giver and receiver of a polarity session. Polarity's life-force is a multilevel concept that explains the source of similar concept, such as India's *prana,* Russian psychic research's "bioplasmic energy," China's *chi* and Yoda's "the Force." It is the energy that animates our body, mind, and spirit so that we truly live, rather than simply exist. Dr. Stone explained this life force and the principles of the Law of Polarity as electromagnetism.

Everything has a positive ($+$), negative ($-$), and neutral (0) charge. Protons, electrons, and neutrons bind atoms and molecules together, giving every cell in the body a charge. This charge attracts or repels, like a magnet. The human cellular low-level magnetism creates a flow of energy throughout and around the body.

Polarity therapists see the body as a core magnet that generates an energy field around it. When we have free-flowing energy, we are like an electromagnet with its current turned on, able to attract what we need and repel what we don't want. Impaired or blocked energy currents begin to shut us down. This body current brownout leaks power and robs us of the ability to take care of ourselves. The physical, mental, emotional, and energetic levels of the body lack the balance and strength to nourish the whole being; stress, pain, and illness result.

Polarity therapy does not identify energy as good or bad, but flowing or blocked. Polarity focuses on the neutral center from which the animating energy emanates, seeking a balance in order to catalyze the client's own healing abilities. It seeks to balance and recharge the flow between positive and negative poles in the body in order to calm nerves, relax muscles, and open natural pathways for the healing force to work. The practitioner places her hands on certain parts of the body, designated as positively or negatively charged. The left hand is negatively charged; the right, positively. In most "polarity positions," the giver places the negative left hand at a positive place on the receiver's body; the positive right on a negative pole. Giver and receiver connect. The client, like a battery, recharges from the freeing up and running of her own energy during the session.

Formal polarity theory diagrams a hierarchy of energy fields and currents. The interaction of the three energies $(+, -, 0)$ create five elements—ether, air, fire, water, and earth—which relate to five chakras and energy currents in the body. These include five vertical currents that correspond to the five elements of Ayurvedic medicine. The five fingers and toes each carry an elemental current.

Actually, polarity recognizes many more currents in the body. The palm of the right hand has a plus $(+)$ charge; the left a minus $(-)$; the head is a positive pole and the feet are negative poles. Connecting the primary currents is seen as more effective and the effects are felt more quickly. However, placing hands on any two parts of the body, exchanging energy between positive and negative poles, will also create an effect.

Another key principle in polarity is that energy manipulation by touch is not enough. Adjustments made in the current flow will not last if poor habits are maintained—in nutrition, exercise, and thought. Food is a collection of energy particles, broken down by the digestive system so cells can absorb the energy as nutrients, joining the body's energy flow. Polarity classifies foods using the five elements of Ayurvedic medicine. The polarity diet and nutrition theory is designed to balance lacking or over-abundant elements.

Exercise is another piece of the total approach. Stone created his own polarity yoga from a number of traditions he studied. His form of exercise is designed to stimulate and release energy, rejuvenating every cell with the life force. Polarity yoga is a series of easy stretching postures which Stone recommended to be practiced for short periods, several times a day.

Finally, all this focus on body energy needs the support of positive thinking. According to Dr. Stone (and various spiritual traditions) thoughts are vibrations of energy that move faster than light or sound. Thoughts and emotions as vibrations affect the flow of energy in the body.

Organs and fluid systems react to highly charged emotions and thoughts. Muscles constrict in unconscious isometrics. Anger held in the gut interrupts energy flow and can lead to lower back pain, sciatica, or other problems. And stress reactions can have effects beyond the physical, sapping the body's energy reserves and its ability to balance and heal itself.

Polarity's point of view includes the ability to revitalize our physical self at will through proper use and control of the mind. Like a self-fulfilling prophecy, if we think we are sick, somehow our actions or the flow impaired by this thought ensures that we become sick. Dr. Stone urged discipline over attitudes and use of positive thought to choose to be healthy.

What Happens in a Polarity Session?

Some polarity techniques are fairly simple and easy to use on friends and family. They can be done on the floor, in a chair, or on a massage table. The comfort of the giver of the bodywork is important, however. The more relaxed and energetically open the doer is, the better the energy flow and exchange during a session.

A polarity session by a practitioner can be a onetime or irregular occurrence but often is part of a series of appointments. A general session is for balancing all of the body's energies. It usually starts at the top with various Head Cradles, then the polarity therapist gently stretches the neck and loosens the shoulders by alternatively pushing each one down toward the feet. The therapist can choose a number of techniques to balance torso energies. He usually does the extremities before having you turn over onto your stomach. In other sessions, the practitioner will start working on specific areas of need.

Most sessions include a basic chakra balancing. The chakras are an East Indian conceptualization of the energy centers at nerve plexuses (intersections) that run up the spine to the top of the head. Polarity connects the first five plexuses, representing its five elements. The practitioner grasps the back of the neck with one hand (the fifth or ether chakra) and places the other hand on the first or earth (coccyx) center. The hand at the back of the neck remains while the other hand works up to the fourth center at the back of the heart area. Sessions usually close with more work on the head and neck and a final "brushing off." The practitioner has you sit up while he sweeps energy down and off your back. I have used just this technique on colleagues at the office to help them to relax and refocus on work.

Applications and Cautions

Polarity can be used to help counteract specific imbalances or conditions. The therapy supports the healing process by promoting three actions—cleansing, building, and toning—on both the physical and energetic levels. There are techniques for certain parts of the body, organs, and systems. Balancing and stimulating the stomach and large intestine aids digestion and elimination. These techniques are handy for relieving indigestion or constipation. The diaphragm positions are not only effective for respiratory and nervous conditions—they've stopped my hiccups!

The chakra balancing technique, the hands-on therapy that sends energy flowing evenly through the plexuses, from tailbone to crown of head, is very relaxing. It is a good general energy toner that balances—not opens up—these power centers and can relieve headaches, stress, tension, and nervousness. Several of the neck techniques can help relax neck tension and move a sore throat through its healing course faster.

There are a number of liver balancing positions, including connecting the liver reflexes, spots similar to acupressure meridian points, just above the elbows and knees. Polarity and Reflexology have a number of foot, hand, and body reflexes in common (see Reflexology).

Polarity also classifies certain organs and conditions by elements. An overactive fire element may activate the stomach, causing sudden hunger. On the other hand, catalyzing the fire element by holding the fire finger and fire toe (the middle ones) stimulates a sluggish liver. Balancing liver functioning affects both nutrient absorption and toxin elimination.

One of the trademark polarity techniques is the *liver flush*, a dietary approach to clearing the liver so it can do its job detoxifying and nourishing the body. The liver flush includes drinking fresh squeezed lemon juice mixed with cold-pressed olive oil and two small cloves of crushed garlic. You take this on an empty stomach first thing in the morning, followed by a special herbal tea (made of ginger, fenugreek, flaxseed, comfrey root, and peppermint), and then fast until lunchtime. When I do a liver flush on workdays, I skip the garlic or use deodorized garlic capsules!

The citrus and oil stimulate the liver and gallbladder to release the toxins, waste, and bile they have been storing for elimination through the large intestines. Some people add a pinch of cayenne pepper. I soften the astringent taste of lemon with grapefruit juice; orange juice is not as effective. I'm usually not hungry until lunch, and after three mornings of "flushing," my digestion feels light and strong.

Polarity is simple, the touch light, and the energy balancing relaxing. Most of the cautions about polarity are the classics. Pregnant women should avoid any technique that stimulates downward energy flow, especially in the abdominal area. While "energy work" is often a good adjunct to many healing programs, it is not a primary treatment for acute or serious medical conditions. However, a number of chiropractors, M.D.s, naturopathic physicians, osteopathic physicians, as well as massage therapists, nurses, counselors, and physical therapists incorporate the polarity philosophy and principles into their practices.

You are the only one who can decide if any dietary or exercise recommendation is comfortable, appropriate, and effective for you. Check it out with your primary care provider if you have any questions. Polarity uses fasting and colonics to clean out the digestion-elimination plumbing in the body. Both of these activities require careful consideration and a call to your primary care provider if you have never done them before.

READ MORE ABOUT IT

POLARITY THERAPY

Health Building: The Conscious Art of Living Well
by Randolph Tone, D.O., D.C.
(Sebastopol, CA: CRCS Publications, 1985)

Your Healing Hands: The Polarity Experience
by Richard Gordon
(Santa Cruz: Unity Press, 1978)

Polarity Therapy
by Alan Siegal, N.D.
(San Leandro, CA: Prism Press, 1987)

Polarity Therapy: The Complete and Collected Works, Vol. I & II
by Dr. Randolph Stone, D.C., D.O.
(Sebastopol, CA: CRCS Publications, 1987)

RESOURCES

American Polarity Therapy Association
P.O. Box 44-154
West Sommerville, MA 02144
(617) 776-6696
❏ information
❏ publication
❏ directory
❏ membership
❏ conference

Reflexology

What Is Reflexology?

Reflexology is a specific bodywork technique of stroking or applying pressure to one part of the body in order to effect changes in another part of the body, relax muscles, and stimulate the body's own natural ability to heal itself.

Reflexology is an American refinement of Oriental wisdom. Like many healing arts, it traces its roots back to Chinese medical philosophy and a theory of energy meridians. There are several techniques lumped under the generic term Reflexology.

❏ hand reflexology

❏ foot reflexology

❏ zone therapy

❏ body reflexology

Reflexologists see a map of the body on the soles of the feet and palms of the hands. Massaging these extremities sends an energy signal that stimulates reflexes, automatic nerve impulses connected to specific areas of the body. Other parts such as the head, ears, torso, and back also contain reflexes corresponding to the whole of the body.

History and Development of Reflexology

Massaging the feet, hands, and body to affect internal organs and muscles has long been a basic technique of Traditional Chinese Medicine, as well as other ancient Oriental healing systems. It was Dr. William Fitzgerald, an American ear, nose, and throat specialist, who introduced this concept to the U.S. around 1913 as Zone Therapy. He divided the body into ten zones, from the head down to the toes and out to the fingers. He taught that the body's bioelectrical energy, known as *chi* in China and *prana* in India (see Acupressure or Acupuncture for further explanation) flowed through these zones to reflex points in the feet and hands. His theory of energy differs from the Chinese theory, which sees the energy circulating along specific pathways, called meridians. However, both theories base their techniques on the same principle of a life force that can be manipulated and enhanced through touch.

In the 1940s, another American, Eunice D. Ingham, further refined Fitzgerald's ideas, concentrating on the feet. Most teachers of reflexology trace their training back to Ingham. Reflexology has since widened its horizons to include hand and body reflexology, though the foot diagram remains the most commonly known form. As the practice spreads to other Western nations, variations on techniques and theory continue to develop.

A British naturopath created an interesting variation in the 1960s, the Metamorphic Technique. Dissatisfied with his general nature cure practice and curious about how life stresses cause illness, Robert St. John explored reflexology. He created his own chart of foot reflex points, superimposing the spine on the inside edge of each foot, from toe to heel.

As he observed the psychological effects of his foot massage treatments, he concluded that the spinal points correlated to the nine months we spent growing in the womb. The spinal reflexes have stored up the emotional traumas we experienced in utero—the negative reaction, for example, that our fetal body experienced when our mothers argued with our fathers, sending a rush of hormones through her system. The Metamorphic Technique aims to smooth out those prenatal imprints or fears that may be causing behaviors or emotional stresses that contribute to ill health.

Reflexology uses foot massage to effect physiological changes which then may have psychoemotional benefits. The Metamorphic Technique uses foot massage to effect psychoemotional changes to reduce physical stress and eliminate illness. This development from the physical (reflexology) to the emotional and spiritual realms (metamorphic) is an illustration of the body-mind-spirit continuum so central to the holistic philosophy.

How Does Reflexology Work?

Zone therapists and reflexologists say that massaging certain points on the body loosens tensions or blockages that stop universal life energy from circulating freely in the body. Free-flowing energy helps the body regain its natural balance, harmony, and health. Reflexology stimulates blood circulation to nourish the body and stimulates the lymph system to cleanse it.

One scientific explanation for how reflexology works is that compressing the skin and tissue just below the skin stimulates sensory receptors. This stimulus telegraphs its message along the afferent ("conducting inward") fibers of the peripheral (outer) nervous system to the spinal cord. The theory states that this stimulation may then disperse through the central and automatic nervous system, producing various effects in any area or zone connected via the spinal cord.

Regardless of the exact method, reflex massage does dilate or constrict the blood vessels, relax or stimulate voluntary muscle contraction, and possibly sedate or stimulate pain in areas remote from the part that is being touched. The principle is similar to acupressure and acupuncture. Relaxing and stimulating the body can help sluggish glands and organs to regain normal functioning. Little "crystals" felt in the foot can be lactic acid, a sediment that settles in your body from poor eating habits or lack of proper exercise. These can be gently crushed and reabsorbed by the body. The lymph systems can then eliminate the waste product.

What Happens in a Reflexology Session?

A masseuse can use reflexology by itself or with several other healing arts. It can be a first aid measure for temporary relief of headaches or a regular routine of self-care. Eclectic massage technicians use reflexology to work on your feet (and hands), combined with other massage techniques to work the rest of the body. My favorite health spa in Calistoga, California, requires its masseuses and masseurs to know acupressure, reflexology, and Swedish massage—three different massage techniques that work different levels and parts of the body in different ways.

Reflexology is simple and easy to learn to do on yourself or a friend. A reflexology massage starts with the masseuse "getting to know" the feet or hands, gently stroking or kneading them as a warm-up. You may be sitting with your feet extended or lying on a table or the floor. Just make sure you are comfortable. A good foot massage can put you out like a light and you don't want to wake up with a stiff neck.

The masseuse holds each foot, using thumbs, mainly, to stroke or press the bottom, top, and sides. You may feel tender spots or little crystals that send a feeling like you're being nipped when they're rubbed too hard. Don't hesitate to say "ouch" to let the messeuse know that it hurts—and say "stop" if it hurts too much. When the masseuse hits one of those painful points, she may hold it for a minute and then go back to it several times until the tenderness recedes. The pressure should be just before or only to the point of pain. We tend to tense up to prevent feeling pain and the point of a massage is relaxation!

There may or may not be a prescribed pattern of massage. Some reflexologists have a routine, some don't. Some use just their hands, others may use a comb, a clothespin, or an elbow to work a particular area or spot. If you have a specific complaint, such as a headache, the masseuse may go over the entire foot or hand first and then concentrate on more points relating to the head. Manipulating parts of the big toe affects the head and neck; other parts of the head are relieved by pressing on the pads just below various toes.

Different versions of reflexology use different maps of the feet. The sinus can be on the big toe on one map, the baby toe on another, and the third toe on yet another. When I asked about the discrepancy, I was actually told that somebody had copyrighted his diagrams, so any subsequent maps have to show some differences when published. It's also possible, say several long-time reflexologists, that different people have different maps or reflex locations on their feet. You may have to experiment for yourself.

The bottom of the foot has the more effective reflex points but working the top and sides of the foot also has benefits. If you are doing this for yourself or a friend, press points for several seconds or minutes, or stroke the foot or hand slowly or rhythmically. Go with what feels good.

Applications and Cautions

Reflexology, like acupressure and acupuncture, is more successful with functional disorders and simple acute conditions than with emergencies. It is recommended for chronic conditions such as asthma, headaches and migraines, constipation, sinus trouble, and stress. This technique does not fix structural problems, such as a hernia, broken bones, or an obstruction of the bowels. However, regular use has a general toning effect which enhances other treatments, and one's vitality and feelings of well-being.

There are few contraindications, but they are ones to heed. Stimulating circulation or energy may accelerate the spread of infection and other conditions compromised by increased circulation.

Once when I went to a Calistoga spa for an enzyme bath and massage to help ward off a cold, Debra (my favorite masseuse) barely touched my feet. She did not want to accelerate the lymphatic system's sloughing off of mucus. A cold is the body's way of ridding itself of waste products. With a virus to fight, it doesn't need the excess baggage of mucus in the lungs, sinuses, or the lymph system. Working the foot reflexes stimulates the blood and lymph glands, increasing circulation and the cleansing process. Dumping too much mucus too fast is like a bad cold, which can knock you out if it is too intense.

Finally, while you may be curious about which areas of the body correspond to a sore point on the foot or hand, the crystals or tenderness you feel may not necessarily be an indication of an illness or compromised organ. The purpose of the reflexology session is to relax the body and enhance its own ability to regain health. The soreness may be sending a message to pay better attention to your health or your body. It's up to you to judge whether you are suffering from the simple effects of an unwise indulgence (those late-night snacks that settle as crystals in your feet) or from something more serious. You need to decide whether to seek the advice of your primary care provider.

READ MORE ABOUT IT

REFLEXOLOGY

Hand and Foot Reflexology: A Self-Help Guide
by Kevin and Barbara Kunz
(New York: Prentice Hall Press, 1984/1987)

Body Reflexology
by Mildred Carter
(West Nyack, NY: Parker Publishing, 1983)

Mirror of the Body
by Anna Kaye and Don C. Matchan
(San Francisco: Strawberry Hill Press, 1978)

Hand Reflexology: Key to Perfect Health
by Mildred Carter
(West Nyack, NY: Parker Publishing, 1975)

The Metamorphic Technique: Principles and Practice
by Gaston Saint-Pierre and Debbie Boater
(Tisbury, Wiltshire, England: Element Books, 1983)

Zone Therapy
by Anika Bergson and Vladimir Tuchak
(Los Angeles: Pinnacle Books, 1974)

Helping Yourself with Foot Reflexology
by Mildred Carter
(West Nyack, NY: Parker Publishing, 1969)

RESOURCES

International Institute of Reflexology
P.O. Box 12462
St. Petersburg, FL 33733
(813) 343-4811
❏ classes
❏ publications
❏ referrals

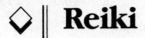# Reiki

What Is Reiki?

Reiki is an energy healing system based on ancient Tibetan knowledge rediscovered by a Japanese theologian. Reiki sessions, performed by practitioners initiated through energy attunement by a Reiki Master, channel Universal Life Energy to family members, friends, or clients. Reiki practitioners transmit this energy by a light touch, a gentle placing of hands in specific positions on the body. Reiki can be used for mental, emotional, physical, or spiritual balancing.

History and Development of Reiki

Reiki's ecumenical approach to healing started with the rediscovery of ancient healing practices by a Japanese Christian in the mid-1800s. Dr. Mikao Usui, a minister in Kyoto, Japan, began researching world religions for a description and understanding of the healing methods of Jesus. Eventually he learned Sanskrit to read the *sutras,* ancient books of esoteric religious teachings. Finally, after years of study and meditation, he recovered the healing knowledge he sought, hidden in the cryptic language and symbols of sacred Tibetan texts.

Usui named this healing system *reiki* from the Japanese words *rei* (boundless and universal) and *ki* (vital life force energy that flows through all living beings). He spent most of the rest of his life wandering, healing the poor, and teaching his method to a few students.

One of his advanced students ran a successful Reiki clinic in Tokyo until World War II. Dr. Jujiro Hyashi, the second Grand Master in the line of tradition after Usui, initiated a Japanese-American woman who eventually imported Reiki back to her home state of Hawaii. Hawayo Takata had come to Japan in the

1930s seriously ill. She found help at Hyashi's clinic and stayed on to train in the Reiki tradition. Takata returned to her home in Hawaii before the war broke out and succeeded Hyashi as Grand Master of the line upon his death in 1941.

For 30 years, Takata kept a low profile as a Reiki healer, finally training and initiating other Reiki masters, starting in the 1970s. Before her death in 1981, she founded the American Reiki Association in order to train more Reiki masters and practitioners. The tradition is now carried on by two worldwide organizations led by students of Takata.

The American International Reiki Association (AIRA) is headed by an American classicist, Dr. Barbara Ray. This group calls Reiki the "Radiance Technique" and has copyrighted the phrase "The Official Reiki Program." It collects case studies to document the Radiance Technique's uses and publishes a journal. Ray is said to have been initiated by Takata to the seventh degree—Reiki's highest level, akin to a black belt in karate—and is therefore able to initiate Masters or teachers to and beyond the third degree.

The Reiki Alliance's Grand Master is Takata's granddaughter, Phyllis Lee Furumoto, who holds to the traditional teachings. You can recognize Alliance members by the phrase "Traditional Usui System of Natural Healing." Both groups have a total of more than 20,000 members or students initiated at least to the first level throughout Europe, Australia, New Zealand, and the U.S.

The AIRA cautions in its literature that some people using the term and symbols of "Reiki" are not fully empowered or appropriately initiated in the system, especially to teach beyond the first two degrees. Ultimately it is up to you, the consumer, to decide for yourself: Are you getting what you want and need for your own self-help or health care goals?

How Does Reiki Work?

Reiki practitioners are the first to say that they don't *exactly* know how it works. Explanations to clients vary from describing it as a relaxation response to showing an energy model, complete with planes of vibrational energy and levels of consciousness. Initiation in this "energy science" means that a Reiki Master links a student to a cosmic, radiant energy, opens *chakras,* or "attunes" that individual as a receiver for Universal Life Energy vibrations or unconditional love.

This series of "attunements" or "empowerments" seems reminiscent of Tibetan Buddhism's ritual empowerments, meant to move devotees closer to enlightenment, except the Reiki systems claim no particular spiritual practice, discipline, or faith requirements. It strikes me as a secularization of an ancient, sacred healing knowledge, partially revealed and adapted for modern times for healing and self-healing.

Most students take the first and second degree initiations, attunements that empower them to share energy in "hands-on sessions." The Usui System says that the first degree training or attunement is for physical healing, the second degree for mental healing plus amplification of the initiate's energy. Sessions can last several minutes or hours. Most regular sessions are an hour.

The Reiki energy is drawn in and focused through the hands to make a link between two living beings. Initiates may say that they shift into a degree level to tap into the energy that is always around us, or that initiation expands the radiant energy within them and that they then focus it through their hands. The higher the degree of initiation, the more power available to channel. One Reiki teacher describes the connection as "lighting up" and energy flowing to balance vibrations. Reiki work is applied to oneself, plants and animals, and even absent people. Absentee healing is a second degree skill or empowerment.

There should be nothing conscious or willful about the process. The energy follows its own laws, going where it seems to be needed despite the intention of the giver or the request of the receiver. Reiki students do a session as meditation with no focus except to offer the flow of energy, expectations set aside.

What Happens in a Session?

Reiki is a relaxing and meditative experience. Clients usually start with a series of three or four full treatments lasting about an hour each. Hands are held in 12 basic positions, each held for five minutes. However, there are many other hand positions possible, and a practitioner may allow intuition to guide them. Holding time is doubled for particular problem areas.

Different people experience Reiki in different ways. The experience can range from feeling more calm and centered to more energized—or both! One of my sessions, given by Radiance teacher Michael O'Leary, was so relaxing, I "went away" in a hypnotic state, a meditative place that is neither asleep nor awake. I also remember feeling more and more warmth radiating from his hands.

Applications and Cautions

Reiki masters and their literature assure the consumer that Reiki is a pure and passive practice of expanding or channeling energy. The Universal Energy comes through and into the receiver or the receiver expands to meet that higher cosmic level.

The one question or concern I have about any energy work or bodywork practice is: How do we, the "uninitiated," know what kind of energy is coming through during a session or a connection? We have not developed new scientific techniques to investigate or judge them, or the mystic vision to see what really transpires when two living beings touch, making an energy connection.

There are times that I do not work on friends or don't want somebody else to work on me because something doesn't feel quite right with one or both of us. So with Reiki, Psychic Healing, Therapeutic Touch, or any healing art, intuition must be your guide. Does this energy experience, this practitioner feel right for you?

Reiki or the Radiance Technique can be applied to anybody or any condition to enhance a treatment program, help relieve pain, or as a general energy "tune-up." Most Reiki practitioners are careful not to promise specific results or relief of symptoms beyond the benefits of relaxation and stress reduction. Anecdotal evidence or testimonics to Reiki's benefits, however, are full of unexpected effects and cures, sped-up healing time, and a few miracles.

One woman taped her hand to her abdomen each night for weeks to relieve abdominal cramps. The pain eventually subsided but first a nearby mole fell off—testimony to the healing energy having its own agenda. Others use Reiki to relieve dental pain. One of my friends had a jaw ache that quickly escalated into an abscessed tooth; the Reiki energy treatment brought a simmering healing crisis to a boil.

O'Leary, a fourth degree Radiance Technique teacher, says

that this energy work can help the terminally ill. It is not so much to cure the cancer, for example. Sometimes there is just "not enough wholeness to expand to sustain physical life," he explains. But the technique can lend mental and emotional support and healing which improve the quality of the time left.

Of course, the usual caveats about not treating pathological conditions solely with an energy treatment apply to Reiki. Get the broken leg set, the high blood pressure regulated, or the migraine diagnosed before or along with the supportive Reiki treatments.

Reiki proponents promote energy work as a complement to a long list of other traditional and modern health care systems. Among those often mentioned are Chiropractic, Homeopathy, Polarity, Massage, Acupressure, Acupuncture, Trager, and the Alexander Technique (see individual chapters). As an energy work, Reiki does not compete with the individual techniques but adds an extra level of energy to the touch of whoever is practicing these other forms of health care.

READ MORE ABOUT IT

REIKI

Reiki: Universal Life Energy
by Bobo J. Baginski and Shalila Sharamon
(Mendocino, CA: Life Rhythms, 1988)

The "Reiki" Factor (expanded edition)
by Barbara Ray, Ph.D.
(St. Petersburg, FL: Radiance Association, 1988)

RESOURCES

American-International Reiki Association
2201 Wilshire Boulevard, Suite 831
Santa Monica, CA 90403
(213) 394-6220
❏ information
❏ publications
❏ referrals

Reiki Alliance
East 33135 Canyon Road
Cataldo, CO 83810
(208) 682-3514

Relaxation Techniques

What Are Relaxation Techniques or Exercises?

Relaxation techniques are just that: methods to help you relax. There are many. Some help you relax your mind; others work primarily on the body. A few see themselves as integrated systems for body-mind-spirit harmony. Some focus on complete muscular relaxation, others promote concentration, while some also increase sensory awareness, all in the name of relaxation. It is up to you to find and choose the style that fits your needs and tastes.

Most of the following methods help you consciously relax muscles and balance your metabolism. Scientifically speaking, you can bring some of your autonomic functions under your voluntary control. Using words, breath, sound, or visual images, these structured methods help you focus on attending to body sensations or thoughts, or on cultivating specific emotional states. The following are some well-known and formalized relaxation techniques:

- ❏ Autogenic Training*
- ❏ Biofecdback*
- ❏ Biogenics
- ❏ Imagery or Visualization
- ❏ Isolation or Flotation Tank (sensory deprivation)
- ❏ Mediation techniques
- ❏ Progressive Relaxation
- ❏ Relaxation Response

255

❏ Systematic Desensitization Therapy

❏ Yoga*

History and Development of Meditation and Relaxation Techniques

Meditation and yoga are relaxation techniques that have been with us since ancient days. Christian, Jewish, and Eastern religious traditions all include some type of meditation, usually associated with their respective mystical traditions, often thought of as prayer. Fourteenth-century Christian literature refers to withdrawing from ordinary consciousness in order to contact God.

The Byzantine church developed a mystical meditation using a repetitive prayer called "The Prayer of the Heart" or "The Prayer of Jesus." Like TM and other meditation techniques, this prayer was found to induce in the follower an altered state, a secret meditation passed on by initiation rite. The Cabalistic tradition, Jewish mysticism, had its contemplative prayers; for example, meditation on the Hebrew letters of God's name, focusing on an image or sound. Relaxation of the body was a by-product of focusing the mind on God.

Sitting Zazen is the centuries-old Zen Buddhist meditative practice. Yoga is the Indian Hindu equivalent. Japanese Shintoism has a practice similar to the Buddhist tradition. American Indian and other shamanic religions use music, drums, or chanting to induce altered states—some more manic than others. Western adaptation of shamanic rituals for visualizations can also be very relaxing and inspiring.

It wasn't until this century that the researchers got into the act and made a science of relaxing. Edmund Jacobson, the grandfather of relaxation techniques, began working at Harvard in 1908. His research led him to conclude that tension caused muscle fibers to shorten. Such tension, he found, was present in people reporting anxiety. If complete absence of muscle contraction is the direct opposite of tension, relaxing muscle tension could eliminate the anxiety, he reasoned. Jacobson published his

---

*See separate chapters

landmark *Progressive Relaxation* in 1929. By the time he died 30 years later, his work had led to a routine of tensing, relaxing, and attending the sensation for each of 15 muscle groups. The training took 56 one-hour sessions.

Joseph Wolpe modified Jacobson's procedures and applied them to a systematic treatment for fears. In 1958, he introduced Systematic Desensitization Therapy. Clients learned to reverse muscle tensing reactions while being exposed to the very thing that they feared.

The '50s also saw John Lilly introduce the isolation tank. The design—a covered tub filled with warm salt-laden water—grew out of his sensory deprivation research for the National Institute of Mental Health. By the '70s, Lilly had refined the flotation tank (sometimes called a "samahdi tank" by meditators who use the tank to bring them closer to a yogic state of union with the Universal Energy) into a popular recreational or meditational relaxation tool. "Floaters" use the tank to change their inner experiences by reducing outer sensory distractions. The movie *Altered States* was an imaginative exaggeration of the mind-expanding potential of such complete isolation.

Meanwhile, back in the '40s, a French cardiologist introduced the benefits of yoga to the Western world. Therese Brosse was the first to attempt documenting the value of meditation in medicine, observing that Indian yogis' activities can affect specific functions of the autonomic nervous systems, such as slowing down the heart rate (see Yoga).

Autogenic Training grew out of the work of German neurologists and psychiatrists and their interest in hypnosis and self-hypnosis, about the same time that Progressive Relaxation was developing in America (see Autogenic Therapy). Patients learned to enter the relaxed body state, similar to being under hypnosis, on their own.

All these threads of mind and body control, muscle and mental relaxation came together with the Greens at the Menninger Foundation, Harvard's Dr. Herbert Benson, and other researchers who have been investigating the abilities of advanced meditators for the past 30 years. Alyce and Elmer Green used electronic measurements to document yogic mastery over automatic body functions such as heart rate and blood pressure previously thought independent (see Biofeedback). The Greens also updated Autogenic Training using electronic machines, calling it Autogenic Biofeedback Training. Along with other biofeedback trainers, they also demonstrated that uninitiated people can learn to control physiological functions, especially for medical and relaxation purposes.

By the '70s, the country was ready for the secularization of meditation. Transcendental meditation (TM) swept the nation on the Beatles' coattails. Benson studied TM, launching a lifelong exploration of the power of meditative discipline. He introduced a similar but nonreligious meditation technique, popularized in his best-seller *The Relaxation Response,* in 1975.

Dr. Norman Shealy has borrowed principles from Autogenics and self-hypnosis, and added life-style changes in diet and exercise for a 90-day self-health program. Biogenics ("origins of life") is a system of mental exercises designed to bring harmony to the body, mind, and spirit. Shealy's goal is a relaxed and physiologically balanced body, a poised and alert mind, and an attuned spirit.

How Do Relaxation Techniques Work?

Stress is the great disrupter of our internal equilibrium, a disturbance in our natural homeostasis. The pressures of modern life and deteriorating environment eat away at our bodies' and minds' ability to heal and function well. Relaxation techniques counteract our stress reactions to the shocks, strains, and pollutants.

A stress reaction is our fight or flight response gone haywire. Herbert Benson calls it an "arousal disorder," where chemical signals from the brain keep flashing "danger." Those chemicals are designed to pump up our heart rate and blood pressure and increase our breathing and the amount of oxygen to the heart and skeletal muscles so we can run from or stand up to whatever danger confronts us.

That was fine when we were struggling to hunt down supper while avoiding becoming a meal ourselves. Today we don't have to attack our enemies like animals. Frustration on the job can trigger the same flood of hormones used to flee a fire. However, anger at work often has nowhere to go. We can end up in a state of constant physiological arousal, muscles tensed and metabolism revved.

Relaxation techniques gear us down to a reasonable speed. Heightened metabolism and muscular tension are consequences of stress responses, unconsciously learned and habituated. Relaxation techniques are designed to help us unlearn the harmful patterns and learn positive habits. They can reduce blood pressure and flow, heart and breathing rate, and hormone levels.

Whether mentally or physically oriented, relaxation techniques generally quiet our "action nerves," our impulse to strike, allowing the body to release tensions both in the mind and in the body. Physiological state changes follow changes in mental-emotional states and vice versa.

The creators of the above-mentioned techniques have written manuals or taught trainers to lay out their specific methods for working. Others have used traditional meditative forms to create a variety of exercises. Almost all relaxation techniques have some common elements.

❑ Quiet environment, few distractions; or, in the case of the isolation tank, near total sensory deprivation.

❑ Restricted attention: the mind is focused on a word, sound, thought, or image—a mental device as a sole stimulus. TM initiates get a secret mantra; shamanic meditation focuses on drumming; modern meditators can purchase a machine that creates "white noise"; or an Eastern meditator might contemplate the Zen koan (riddle) "What is the sound of one hand clapping?" as something to quiet the mind.

❑ Passive attitude: letting go of the effort to *do* it or to do it right. Checking on your performance or demanding a response creates its own tension.

❑ Direct or indirect suggestion to relax.

❑ Comfortable position for unrestricted energy flow or consciously relaxing muscles: loosening tight clothing, lying or sitting to reduce the physical distraction of an uncomfortable position.

I might argue about that regarding sitting Zazen or in a lotus position. However I hear that, like the marathon runner who "hits the wall" and passes through, the physical discomfort is part of the discipline and soon forgotten in reaching meditation's euphoric goals.

Doing Relaxation Techniques

Most relaxation techniques are easily learned, ideal self-help tools. Choosing a good guide or training at the start seems to be the key to a lifetime of benefit. Books, classes, tapes, and videos abound for instruction and practice. A stress reduction class may be a good place to begin learning the exercises. Books and training literature can help you decide which technique interests you.

Some kinds of stress can become a chronic condition which took years to develop. The road back to a balanced and relaxed body is going to be equally long. I would consider exploring a number of techniques until I found one that I could and would do every day. However, you don't have to choose a formal technique to benefit from relaxation exercises.

Various aerobics and meditation teachers taught me their versions of relaxation exercises, most of them adaptations or combinations of elements from the above techniques. Once you get the idea from a time-tested form, it is fun to create one on your own which works for you. You can even make a tape with your favorite music and instructions.

And, lest we forget and think relaxation is only a formal exercise or discipline, humans have managed to find ways to relax before some tried to make a science of it! Some everyday techniques include:

❏ A few deep breaths or breathing exercises

❏ Dancing and other rhythmic movement or exercises

❏ Getting away from it all—a mini or major vacation

❏ Hobbies, such as arts or crafts

❏ Reading, coloring a coloring book, or another quiet activity

❏ Listening to music or playing an instrument

❏ Having a heart-to-heart talk with a grandparent or other wise person

❑ Walking

❑ Prayer

❑ Mud baths (or enzyme baths if you live in Japan or the San Francisco Bay Area)

Applications and Cautions

Stress-related diseases can benefit from the stress-reducing results of these techniques. Relaxation is often the major element in the course of treatment for conditions such as insomnia, peptic ulcer, nervous fatigue, migraine headaches, nail biting, depression, stuttering, premature ejaculation and other sexual disorders.

If you are claustrophobic like me, the flotation tank could scare you off in a minute. But John Lilly's claim of pain relief might inspire me if I were mending a broken leg like he was. It seems the heavy concentration of Epsom salts, the seeming suspension of gravity, and the increased release of endorphins (the body's own painkillers) make flotation effective for relieving intense, chronic pain. And my floater friends remind me that you're not locked in, you can reach up and push open the little door any time.

Many of these techniques are useful adjuncts to psychotherapy, on the advice of the therapist. The resulting sensory awareness, perceptual clarity, memory retrieval, and reduced physical tension can stimulate deeper awareness of repressed emotions and psychological processes.

Herbert Benton's decades of studying meditative techniques reveal two life-enhancing, if not lifesaving, benefits of longtime practice. First is a "Faith Factor" which, when combined with relaxation, enables meditators to reach enhanced states of well-being and health. He found that meditators with deep spiritual beliefs could overcome insomnia, headaches, and panic attacks, as well as enhance cancer therapies.

Second is a mental plasticity he calls the "Principle of Maximum Mind." It opens the mind to new ways of thinking and seeing the world and ourselves. For example, athletes enhance their sports skills with imagery, eliciting the "relaxation response" for optimum performance.

This may be the most profound application of any of these techniques. Whatever we call it—positive thinking, a new view of ourselves, or heightened mental powers—it empowers us to change our lives and is the key to healing ourselves, as well as helping our families, our country, and our planet.

However, profound meditative relaxation may cause some problems. Done to an extreme, one can get too relaxed, one's mind too plastic. Profound relaxation over a prolonged period heightens suggestibility. A plastic mind, when gained in spiritual pursuits, may leave the meditator open to "cultic emanations," Benson warns.

I have also met spiritual seekers with what some of us at JFK University used to call "losing your boundaries" or "Meditation Sickness." On the one hand, deep physiological relaxation can allow the body to release painful emotions and emotional memories. Stimulated too often or too fast, the new emotional awareness may be too intense. The individual becomes one raw nerve, suffering the impact of things and people inordinately in everyday life.

On the other hand, some people may become addicted to the seeming euphoria of relaxation and withdraw from active life—physically and/or emotionally. Meditation or another form of relaxation becomes a shield, a way not to deal with real life.

READ MORE ABOUT IT

RELAXATION TECHNIQUES

Stress and the Art of Biofeedback
By Barbara Brown
(New York: Harper & Row, 1977)

Relax: How You Can Feel Better, Reduce Stress and Overcome Tension
edited by John White and James Fadiman
(The Confusion Press, 1976)

Progressive Relaxation Training: A Manual for the Helping Professions
by Douglas Bernstein and Thomas D. Borkovec
(Champaign, IL: Research Press, 1973)

Progressive Relaxation: A Physiological and Clinical Investigation
by Edmund Jacobson
(Chicago: University of Chicago Press, 1938)

The Relaxation Controversy: Can You Relax Without Meditation?
by Martin Ebon
(New York: New American Library, 1976)

The Book of Floating
by Michael Hutchinson
(New York: Wiliam Morrow, 1984)

RESOURCES

Vippassana Meditation Center
P.O. Box 24
Shelbourne Falls, MA 01370
(415) 625-2160
        or
P.O. Box 510
Occidental, CA 95465
(707) 874-3031
❏ information
❏ retreat center

Insight Meditation Society
Pleasant Street
Barre, MA 01005
(508) 355-4378

Ananda Community
14614 Tyler Foote Road
Nevada City, CA 95959
(916) 292-3494
❏ information
❏ classes
❏ publications
❏ products
❏ speakers
❏ membership
❏ referrals to centers worldwide

Flotation Tank Association
P.O. Box 1396
Grass Valley, CA 95945
(916) 432-3794
❏ publication
❏ membership
❏ referrals

Rolfing

What Is Rolfing or Structural Integration?

Rolfing is a series of ten basic bodywork sessions of deep connective tissue manipulation. It is named after its founder, Ida P. Rolf. She called her system Structural Integration, which described her original goal in creating it. The aim of Rolfing is to increase muscular length and overall balance for optimal posture, as measured along a vertical axis from the ear to the ankle. An aligned body balances better against gravity, allowing the body to use energy more efficiently. In addition, Rolfing Movement Integration applies new postural awareness to everyday actions and activities.

Appropriately, Rolfing therapists are often called Rolfers. Several of Rolf's protégés have used her theories as the basis for their own forms of bodywork. These variations often involve techniques less invasive than Rolfing and focus on the psycho-emotional issues brought forth during the process of physical restructuring.

History and Development of Rolfing and Other Structural Aligning Bodywork Systems

Born in New York in 1896, Rolf earned a Ph.D. in biochemistry from Columbia Unviersity's College of Physicians and Surgeons in 1916. She worked for the Rockefeller Institute (now Rockefeller University) until the late 1920s, when family business forced her to leave. A bright and determined individual, Rolf continued pursuing her interests in a wide variety of medical and health practices.

The seeds of Rolfing were planted when Rolf helped her

childrens' piano teacher recover the use of an injured hand. Rolf taught the woman yoga, believing that the muscle stretching exercises helped the muscles and soft tissue return to optimal length and position in the body. However, in practicing yoga, she realized that the manipulations actually caused some joints to contract. She began to search for other exercises to add to her nascent treatment system.

Rolf explored the ideas of the Alexander Technique and studied osteopathy, incorporating the view that structure determines function. She saw that when one part of the body was troubled, it threw the whole body off balance. Further, a distorted body structure, she learned, inhibits optimal physical functioning. Rolf introduced to her work exercises and manipulations she learned from a California osteopath named Amy Cochran.

By the early 1950s, Rolf was teaching her Structural Integration in the U.S., Canada, and England. However, she was frustrated with the chiropractors and osteopaths who tried to incorporate her system into their own fields as just another technique. They missed the point. Hers was a systemic approach, balancing all parts of the body, rather than, as she put it, "chasing around the body" after individual distortions.

Rolf's big break came when the founder of Gestalt therapy, Fritz Perls, invited her to the Esalen Institute to work on him. A student of Rolf had helped the irrepressible Perls, using Structural Integration techniques, but she felt unqualified to do more because of Perls's serious heart condition. The student told him to go to the source, Ida Rolf.

Rolf spent a week at the mecca of the burgeoning human potential movement, working on Perls and sitting in on his classes. On the last day, the seventh session, Rolf was working on his neck. Perls suddenly became unconscious. Rolf first feared that she had triggered a heart attack, then she noticed that he looked more like someone under anesthesia than someone experiencing cardiac arrest.

A few minutes later, Perls came to and mentioned that he had once been injured by an anesthetist during surgery. Rolf realized that her working on Perls's neck had recalled that memory from his muscles. Release of stored physical or emotional trauma is indeed a common occurrence during Rolfing.

Perls, whose heart condition improved after his Rolfing,

referred to Ida Rolf as "Mrs. Elbows" in his book, *In and Out of the Garbage Pail*. And Rolf began spending summers at Esalen's Big Sur compound, teaching and working on a newly appreciative audience.

Rolf and Rolfing showed up in various articles about Esalen, the human potential movement, and the new "bodywork" treatments. The growing popularity of Rolfing, along with the spreading tales of positive results she achieved with her clients, led to research projects documenting the effects of Rolfing. These experiences showed that Rolfing sessions did result in an increase in muscular efficiency.

Another research experiment in 1969 included a Rolfer and an "aura reader." Monitored both by machines and these two observers, the results confirmed the change in subjects' "energy bodies." The changes in the aura observed by the aura reader corresponded consistently with the changes observed by the Rolfer and the machines. In addition, the aura reader observed that the Rolfer's energy also took on a "healing color" (in this case, blue) within a few minutes after the start of each session.

By 1970, there were 40 trained Rolfers. They organized the Rolfer Institute to free Ida Rolf to write, lecture, and work with advanced students. Modeled as a craft guild and incorporated as a nonprofit educational institution, the Institute continues to train and certify Rolfers. In fact, the training is like a graduate degree, with extensive prerequisites in both physical and psychological studies.

Ida Rolf published her first book describing her healing modality in 1977, *Rolfing: The Integration of Human Structures*. She died in 1979, leaving the Rolf Institute to carry on her work.

A number of Rolf's students and longtime members of the Rolf Institute have gone on to establish their own forms of postural aligning bodywork. Joseph Heller created Hellerwork, a more gentle approach to releasing muscle tissue adhesion. It adds an emphasis on verbal processing of issues and memories that are released during bodywork sessions, and on movement education to increase self-awareness.

Aston Patterning is another offshoot of Rolfing. One of Rolf's top trainees, Judith Aston, differed with her teacher on the use of force and symmetry in working with the body. Aston created her own approach to optimal body structuring and applied it to movement activities, especially sports.

A third human structure and balance-oriented bodywork is Jack Painter's Postural Integration, also called Connective Tissue Polarity. Painter's use of Reichian and Gestalt methods bring this kind of mind/bodywork close to the area of body-oriented psychotherapy. These healing arts distinguish themselves from Rolfing by paying more attention to the psychoemotional effects of physical restructuring than Rolf originally taught.

Finally, while not necessarily stemming from the same developmental roots but quite compatible with Rolfing, is Upledger's CranioSacral Therapy. This extremely gentle hands-on work attempts to release twisted connective tissue and compacted structure by amplifying the body's own natural, internal rhythms. It allows the body to recapture its original or optimum shape through its own energetic urges.

How Does Rolfing Work?

The free flow of energy aids the body's own ability to heal itself. This is a principle stated over and over again, in many different ways, by healing arts from Traditional Chinese Medicine and acupressure to Polarity Therapy and the Rosen Method. Rolfing addresses this principle structurally, by aligning the body so the forces of gravity can flow freely throughout. Rolf saw gravity as an omnipresent, all-powerful, and unremitting determinant of "uprightness," or lack thereof.

Rolf characterized the body as a group of stackable units, structured by bones and soft tissue. Bones hold the body's position in space; soft tissues, including the muscles, tendons, ligaments, and other connecting tissues, hold the bones in position.

Like other structured entities, humans are subject to the laws of mechanics. One law states that masses must be balanced in order to be stable. If muscles are chronically shortened, they pull the attached bones out of balance. Repositioning the bone is not enough; individual tissues need to be lengthened for the realignment to be permanent.

Rolfing is a series of ten hour-long sessions to balance the distribution of weight of the major parts of the body by stretching and lengthening soft tissues. At the end of the process, the head, chest, pelvis, and legs are each evaluated for alignment with one another. An imaginary plumb line is drawn from the ear through the shoulder, the hip, knee, and down to the ankle. When the line is straight, the body can move with more grace and efficiency.

Dr. Valerie Hunt, director of UCLA's Movement Behavior Laboratory, and Dr. Julian Silverman, Research Specialist for the California Department of Mental Hygiene, confirmed these results in experiments at the Agnews State Hospital. They found that after the program of ten Rolfings, subjects had more efficient use of muscles, tended to conserve energy, and had increased refinement of movement response.

What Happens in a Session?

A Rolfing session begins with an evaluation and history-taking. Come prepared to list all injuries, illnesses, surgeries, and major emotional traumas that may contribute to your chronic muscular distortions. The Rolfer will also ask you your goals for Rolfing and take a "before" photo of your body.

The Rolfer looks at you in your underwear from all four sides to see how your major "blocks of weight" are stacked along that imaginary plumb line from ear to ankle. Mine talked to me about what she saw, and the way I seemed to hold my body in a ready-to-move position. Since I already had decades of health-seeking under my belt, I was pleased to hear that I was in pretty good alignment. Still, there was more that Rolfing could do to rebalance me.

The first session starts with gentle abdominal breathing. The Rolfer focuses on releasing the outermost sheath of myofacia (muscle tissue) that lies just under the skin. The session also works on lengthening the trunk up out of the pelvis and the legs down from the hip joint.

Depending on the training and other certification taken by your Rolfer, the actual style of Rolfing may vary from one practitioner to another. Audrey Seymour, for example, a Marin County, California, Rolfer, also practices CranioSacral Therapy. She can be in the middle of a Rolfing session and intuitively know when to stop manipulating tissue. She will pause to hold that part of the body lightly and, in the Upledger technique style, evoke a natural cranial-sacral pulse so the body can work through a muscular distortion of the memory of a past trauma.

I find the CranioSacral work much more to my liking. It is a more evocative healing art, practiced with gentle give-and-take as the practitioner leads your body into releasing and balancing itself. Rolfing is a more interventive technique, with the practitioner directly performing intense, modifying bodywork.

Since its beginning, Rolfing has carried a reputation for being painful. Seymour explains that while Rolfing is still interventive, today it is much less painful than people believe. The client is supposed to be active, moving body parts against the Rolfer's stroke. This pulls the muscle from the inside edge while the Rolfer stretches it from the outside surface. It also gives the client a greater sense of participation and control, always helpful in any potentially painful treatment.

Pain signals that the Rolfer is moving too much tissue, too fast. Some clients may prefer that kind of intensity, however. You can decide if you want or need this painful pace. If not, either you can ask the Rolfer to slow down or you can make sure not to pull against her stroke so much as she works. And, if sometimes it does hurt, Rolfers encourage you to "let it out." You don't have to bear the pain in stoic silence; it's okay to groan and yell.

Applications and Cautions

Most people who come to be Rolfed are uncomfortable in their bodies, or are in some sort of physical pain. Their bodies are distorted in some way—shoulders uneven or hunched, back aching, or legs twisted. Many clients achieve relief from chronic complaints as a by-product of Rolfing. However, Rolf was not particularly interested in addressing specific symptoms. She believed that by aligning the body for free energy flow, the body takes care of itself.

Some "Rolfees" are motivated by potential release of memories and emotions during the sessions. They use Rolfing as an adjunct to psychotherapy, a way to work with their bodies as well as their emotions. Whatever nagging symptoms or chronic conditions they experience, Rolfees tend to be highly motivated. They may have to be because, in effect, they are working to drop a lifelong build-up of muscular armoring.

Armoring is a label created by Wilhelm Reich, a contemporary of Sigmund Freud, for the way we build a bodily barrier for all our physical and psychic wounds in life. Tightened muscles form a wall against the slings and arrows of our hectic and sometimes painful lives.

Rolfing may not always be appropriate. Some people need their armoring. For example, one Rolfer recognized halfway through a first session with a prison guard that this client needed his armor to survive his job. The session was so painful that he quit. In its own wisdom, the man's body was refusing to release the knots and bulges. Though motivated to relieve his pain, this Rolfer realized that the guard was subconsciously choosing backaches as a trade-off for protecting his feelings in a brutal prison environment.

This same Rolfer worked on a psychic who came to understand that she was not yet ready to be Rolfed. This woman realized she needed to learn to create better psychic boundaries between herself and her own clients before she would be able to drop the muscular boundaries that protected her. The Rolf Institute also tells its trainees a story about a prostitute who realized that getting Rolfed was making her too sensitive and vulnerable for her line of work.

Persons with cancer and acute conditions such as osteoporosis also should approach Rolfing with caution. Like other healing arts that stimulate circulation, Rolfing may encourage the spread of a malignancy. And in extreme cases, some older people with brittle bones could suffer a cracked 12th rib from a careless practitioner. Rolfers also are cautious with inflamed or swollen conditions and skin disorders, sometimes working around the injury or just waiting until the swelling has gone down or the skin eruption is healed.

READ MORE ABOUT IT

ROLFING

Ida Rolf Talks about Rolfing and Physical Reality
edited by Rosemary Feitis
(New York: Harper & Row, 1978)

Rolfing: The Integration of Human Structures
by Ida P. Rolf, Ph. D.
(Santa Monica: Dennis-Landman, 1977)

The Protean Body: A Rolfer's View of Human Flexibility
by Don Johnson
(New York: Harper Colophon Books, 1977)

Bodywise
by Joseph Heller and William A. Henkin
(Los Angeles: Jeremy P. Tarcher, 1986)

The Complete Book of Rolfing: Using the New Physical Therapy
    to Restructure Your Life
by Gary W. Reid
(New York: Drake Publishers, 1978)

Craniosacral Therapy
by John E. Upledger, D.O., F.A.A.O. and
    John D. Vredovoogd, M.F.A.
(Seattle: Eastland Press, 1983)

RESOURCES

International Rolf Institute
P.O. Box 1868
Boulder, CO 80306
(303) 449-5903
❏ information
❏ referrals
❏ publications
❏ training and certification

The Aston Training Center
P.O. Box 3568
Incline Village, NV 89450
(702) 831-8228
❏ information
❏ referrals
❏ training and certification
❏ workshops
❏ products

The Body of Knowledge/Hellerwork
415 North Mt. Shasta Boulevard, Suite 4
Mt. Shasta, CA 96067
(916) 926-2500 or (916) 929-BODY
❏ training
❏ referrals

❏ classes
❏ speakers
❏ membership

The Upledger Institute (CranioSacral Therapy)
11211 Prosperity Farms Road
Palm Beach Gardens, FL 33410
(800) 223-5880
❏ publications
❏ classes and trainings
❏ consultations

Rosen Method

 ## What Are Rosen Method Bodywork and Movement?

Rosen Method bodywork combines touch and verbal communication to evoke muscular relaxation. Using light to medium touch to increase body self-awareness, this bodywork focuses on muscular tension, the relationship between that tension and the emotions, and the role of breath in creating more space and flexibility in one's physical structure. Rosen Movement involves gentle range-of-motion exercises set to music.

Created by a San Francisco Bay Area physical therapist, this system approaches the body as a living autobiography in which the muscles, joints, and circulatory system speak of repressed memories and emotions, and give clues about the clients' personal and philosophical ways of dealing with life. The Rosen Method works through these issues, offering the possibility of enhanced psychological and emotional health along with improved body shape and functioning.

History and Development of the Rosen Method

The Rosen Method grew out of the studies and work of a refugee from Nazi Germany in the decades after World War II. Marion Rosen was born in Nuremberg in 1914 to a moderately affluent merchant family.

As a young woman, Rosen was introduced to an intellectual circle of psychotherapists by family friends Lucy and Dr. Gustav H. Heyer. The Heyers were members of a group in Munich that combined massage, breathwork, and relaxation techniques with psychoanalysis. Gustav, a colleague and former student of Carl Jung, handled the talk therapy with each client. His ex-wife, a masseuse and dancer, did the bodywork therapies.

Lucy Heyer was a student of Elsa Gindler, then the leading investigator studying the integration of physical and personal development. Considered the "grandmother" of today's breathing and relaxation techniques, Gindler, in turn, was an associate of Karen Horney, one of the leading theoreticians of modern psychoanalysis.

Raised Lutheran but born a Jew, Rosen was barred from the universities of Nazi Germany. She studied instead as an apprentice to Lucy Heyer, assisting her with the massage and breathing sessions. After completing her training, Rosen fled to Sweden to wait for a visa to America, spending two years observing dance classes and completing her physiotherapy training. She planned to work for Gindler and Horney in New York, but had to travel eastward, arriving in San Francisco first.

After seeing San Francisco, Rosen decided to stay on the West Coast. She spent the war working as a physical therapist, treating injured workers from the shipyards. Rosen took premed classes at U.C. Berkeley and studied advanced physical therapy at the Mayo Clinic. Returning from Minnesota, Rosen opened her private practice in Oakland, which she maintained for the next 40 years.

It was in her day-to-day work with a wide variety of patients that Rosen continued to hone the perspective and techniques that she had begun developing in Munich with the Heyers. She sometimes talked to patients about their ailments, noticing that patients who freely discussed events in their lives at the time of the injury recovered more quickly. Slowly, Rosen put more trust and emphasis on the verbal part of her work. Results were increasingly positive. It took a "Mind Dynamics" seminar, however, to convince Rosen that perhaps she had something special to teach, an entirely new technique.

Rosen took the early Werner Erhard (*est*) seminar after seeing the dramatic improvement it fostered in one of her most difficult patients. The experience further convinced Rosen of the effectiveness of verbal expression or processing, and give her confidence to offer introductory workshops in what is now called the Rosen Method. In the '70s she took on her first apprentices, and in 1980 she began her first professional training. Those early apprentices and certified Rosen practitioners established the Rosen Institute, with Marion Rosen as founder and as a principal-teacher who continues to train certified practitioners. Rosen graduates practice in the U.S., Canada, in Europe, and, most recently, in the Soviet Union. A progressive Swedish group, Axelson's Gymnastiska Institut, conducts Rosen trainings in several European countries.

How Does the Rosen Method Work?

Rosen practitioners focus on allowing the body to give up chronic muscle tension and achieve its own natural shape and functioning. Long-term muscle contractions result in dense and rigid muscle tissue and immobilized joints. This makes the body less spacious, less flexible. Limited mobility also inhibits functioning and expression. Changing somatic (body) habit patterns opens options for fuller movement and greater self-expression.

The Rosen body philosophy says that typical socialization processes have taught us to restrict and repress ourselves. We build a "persona," or mask, that is both emotional and physical. Mental barriers and the repression of authentic feelings, reroute emotional energy into a circuit of tension. The tension keeps the muscles unnecessarily contracted, further inhibiting feelings and emotional expression.

For example, as youngsters we are taught, "Big boys (or girls) don't cry." So we believe that crying is unacceptable self-expression. Children then tighten neck and chest muscles to repress the urge to cry. Eventually not only are feelings numbed, but the tension can stiffen the neck. The chest and shoulders knot up and the individual develops a top-heavy look.

Rosen treatments offer clients the conscious process of gaining awareness of their authentic selves. Touch is used to invite this awareness. Often it is first experienced as pain. The body cries for help and for release, an acknowledgement of imbalances and tension. Awareness often calls up images, thoughts, or emotional feeling tones that may trigger a memory connected to that pain. It invites the choice to relax, to choose whether to withhold or express these feelings.

Rosen practitioners are trained to ask open, nonthreatening questions to help draw out memories of earlier events that may be connected to and contained within the muscle knot. Naming the feeling or the memory can help evoke a release. Rosen believes that whatever comes up in a session is already known to the client. These are memories forgotten, feelings denied. Each session offers an opportunity to give up the need to repress feelings that restrict both the body's healthy functioning and the mind's expression and creativity.

The practitioner uses breath as the indicator of change or release. Rosen teaches that the breath is the intersection between conscious and unconscious processes. She links voluntary breathing to conscious activity; autonomic, or reflex, breathing to unconscious activity. Therefore, breath is the most obvious and available way to measure and observe the mind-body dialogue.

The key is the diaphragm, a dome-shaped muscle that divides the thoracic organs (heart and lungs) from the upper abdominal organs (stomach, spleen, and liver). Flattening down to draw air into the lungs and relaxing back into its natural arch to exhale, the diaphragm massages and tones the organs above and below it.

Chronic tension limits the diaphragm's range of motion and the body's capacity to breathe. In a Rosen session, emphasis is often placed on working the diaphragm and surrounding muscles. As the diaphragm regains its natural range of movement, breathing capacity increases. Oxygen fills the organs and muscles. Changes in breathing patterns also change psychological states and emotional reactions. Deeper breathing allows more depth of feeling and more connection to one's authentic self.

What Happens in a Session?

The practitioner usually begins by doing a formal or informal assessment of the client's body shape and movements. How free or restricted are the limbs? Where are the muscle masses or holdings? What is numb or stiff? What hurts? Are the shoulders even, the buttocks held in, the feet pointing straight ahead?

Rosen Method bodywork is done on a massage table with the client partially clothed. No oils are used. Hands-on work often begins with the back of the diaphragm and surrounding muscle groups. At first, a client's back may only expand minimally with each breath, barely moving from shoulder blades to waistline. As muscles are gently probed and awakened, the breath moves both higher and lower through the body. Muscles from thigh to shoulder move with each breath. The body seems more alive, motile, relaxed. Sometimes Rosen workers will ask what the client is thinking, feeling, or remembering if they see a muscle quiver or the skin suddenly flush before softening.

Breathing can change in rhythm and depth many times throughout a session. A natural deep breath indicates new territory opening up, a release evoked. Sudden restriction in the diaphragm often means that the dialogue has struck an issue or a memory that verges on the edge of the client's conscious awareness.

The practitioner's touch can be light, barely manipulating the muscles. Others penetrate deeper. Chronic muscle tension can be hard as a rock and impervious to a light touch's invitation to sensation or self-awareness. Each practitioner evolves her or his own style of touch and contact.

Rosen has no set procedure. Practitioners act from their observations and intuitions, letting their hands go to where their attention draws them. Clients may talk or not talk.

The Rosen Method approach evokes a sense of mother-infant contact. This bond is a vital factor in creating a feeling of trust and a safe environment for sharing emotions and released memories. In a classroom full of students giving and receiving Rosen sessions, the change in the room's atmosphere is palpable. As each pair reaches a state of mental communion, the silence is tender, caring, and calming. Each massage table becomes its own little island of humanistic healing.

I have taken a series of Rosen sessions and classes over the years. They helped change the shape of my body and the depth of my feelings. I found it a great adjuct to psychotherapy. The sessions aided me in getting in touch with long repressed childhood memories. My three sessions with Marion Rosen herself were profound. Like many of the originators of healing modalities or techniques, she has a special genius. During each session, she zeroed in on a deeply buried incident, helping me draw out the memory and understand the defensive decision I had made not to feel the accompanying emotions.

The release of muscular barriers, joined by many painful tears, reshaped my back and chest. My shoulders now are not quite so high around my ears, nor rounded forward in an unconscious effort to protect my young heart. Still something of a klutz at times, I am much more balanced in my movements, and less restricted when I talk and walk.

Applications and Cautions

Rosen work is both stand-alone bodywork and an excellent adjunct to psychotherapy. Born out of Rosen's work with German researchers integrating psychoanalysis and massage-breathwork, the training fosters a deep understanding of the body-mind unity, especially in therapeutic applications.

The release of habitual muscle tension and the triggering of related memories bring out the feelings and emotions to be covered in the talk-therapy. The verbal aspect of the Rosen Method can help clients sort out common life issues. If psycho-emotional problems are severe, however, clients are referred to psychotherapy.

Several Rosen practitioners specialize in working with recovering alcoholics, chemical or process addicts, co-dependents (those in relationships with addicts), and adult children of alcoholics. The gentle, evocative nature of the work makes it an ideal complement to the self-help and therapeutic support most of these individuals seek in recovery.

The releasing-relaxing effects of this method are also good for the body's functioning and immune system. Chronic muscle tension restricts blood and lymph circulation. Denied full oxygenation, muscles underperform. And inefficient cellular waste removal leaves them vulnerable to fatigue and pain.

Rosen work stimulates the parasympathetic nervous system, whose functions include the constriction of the pupils and the slowing of the heartbeat. Circulation is increased. Warmth and color return to areas once frozen in fear or pain. Improved circulation, in turn, increases range of movement. Mobilized joints allow more synovial fluid to lubricate and nourish surrounding cartilage and connective tissues. The gentle Rosen Movement is ideal for seniors.

READ MORE ABOUT IT

ROSEN METHOD

Rosen Method: An Approach to Wholeness and Well-Being Through the Body
by Elaine L. Mayland, Ph.D. (Self-Published/Palo Alto; Berkeley: Rosen Institute, 1984/1988)

The Body Has Its Reasons: Anti-Exercise and Self-Awareness
by Therese Bertherat and Carol Berstein (New York: Avon, 1976/1979)

The Thinking Body: A Study of the Balancing Forces of Dynamic Man
by Mabel E. Todd (Brooklyn, NY: Dance Horizons, 1937)

RESOURCES

Rosen Institute
2315 Prince Street
Berkeley, CA 94702
(415) 548-1205
❏ information
❏ classes
❏ referrals
❏ consultations
❏ trainings and certification

Shamanism

What Are Shamanic Medicine and Neo-Shamanism?

Shamanism is an early spiritual and medical tradition still practiced in native cultures around the globe. Based on the belief that all healing includes the spiritual dimension, shamans enter altered states of consciousness to communicate with other realms of reality. The traditional shaman takes this "journey" to help the patient or community rediscover their connections to Nature and the Divine.

Neo-Shamanism adapts shamanic techniques for holistic healing and encompasses a growing awareness of our responsibility toward nature. A major feature is the fostering of individuals' direct contact with their spirit guides, rather than contact through the shaman. Neo-shamanism also draws on shamanic medicine's adept use of ritual and psychology for therapeutic applications.

History and Development of Shamanism and Neo-Shamanism

Shamanic medicine is an old tradition of knowledge dating back thousands of years. The first healers were responsible for both the health of the individuals in their tribe and for the well-being of the community. Health is physical, mental, emotional, and spiritual balance. Sickness could be a sign of family, clan, or tribal disharmony, as much as a person's own ills.

These tribal priest/healers were our first wise ones, ritual leaders, dream interpreters, herbalists, and mediators between the everyday and spirit worlds. As hunting and gathering and fishing tribes settled into villages, the role of the shaman changed, splitting religion from medicine. Priests took over the religious rituals, shamans the healings. However, shamans still used ritual and magic as part of their lore.

Some cultures specified the shamanic role even further. Sorcerers and witches sold cures, spells, and hexes. Curanderos and curanderas were the herbal healers while sabias and sabios are "wise ones," the sages of the tribes in South or Central America.

Shamanic traditions are similar around the world; but, as Western anthropologists report, different aspects are emphasized in different cultures. Southern Hemisphere tribal societies believed in sorcery or voodoo, the spirit-caused illnesses. Trance healing is still widespread in South America, as is the use of hallucinogens. Tribes in Australia, the Pacific Islands, and South America practice sucking out the disease object, a forerunner to the psychic surgery popular in the Philippines. North American Indians focused on herbal traditions and elaborate healing ceremonies. In fact, much of the early knowledge that inspired the herbal medicine movement in the U.S. came from Westerners who studied various tribal medicine practices.

The influence of shamanism pervades history and the world's religions. Tibetan Buddhism's *bardos,* or planes of existence after death, parallel shamanic spirit worlds. Meditation mandalas are similar to sand paintings or mesa tables used for healing ceremonies. Mantras, like drumming, summon altered states.

Michael Harner, anthropologist and author of *The Way of the Shaman,* proposes that yoga evolved from the need for city-dwelling shamans to hide their spiritual practices. Shamanism had become a dangerous practice when it began to threaten the dominance of state religions' and governments' monopoly on spiritual knowledge. Drumming and chanting would betray the shaman's ritual. Silent meditation techniques to change levels of consciousness more quietly may have eventually developed into the poses and mindfulness of yoga.

Practitioners of such shamanic rituals as divination, prophecy, and herbal medicine were persecuted as witches in the eighteenth-century Western world. But parts of these and related native traditions have survived in today's "occult sciences," such as alchemy, psychic or faith healing, and ritual magic.

Most important, the respect of shamanic and native cultures for nature and Mother Earth inspire our current ecology movements. Shaminism teaches us that our responsibility is to "walk in balance," to live harmoniously with nature. The idea of people as caretakers of the earth is slowly seeping into modern global awareness and politics.

Native shamans are breaking the silence and sharing sacred and powerful knowledge with a wider audience. It started with anthropologists Carlos Castaneda and Harner, followed by Lynn Andrews. They turned their apprenticeship experiences (real or professed) with medicine men and women into a series of popular visionary books and seminars. Frank Water's *The Book of the Hopi* added fuel to the growing interest in native American culture, spiritualism, and prophecy. Spiritual seekers have added terms like *medicine wheel, sweat lodge, power animals, prayer pipe,* and *shamanic state of consciousness* to their lexicons.

Hundreds flock to the weekend Medicine Wheel Gatherings with Sun Bear, a Chippewa medicine man and former Hollywood actor, and the Bear Tribe to pray, cleanse the body and mind, and rediscover their connection to the spirit. A Medicine Wheel is a ceremonial circle used to celebrate our connection to 36 elements of the universe, including animals, Grandmother Moon and Grandfather Sun, love and trust.

Parapsychologist Stanley Krippner and anthropologist Albert Villoldo study shaman/healers such as Rolling Thunder, a railroad brakeman and Cherokee medicine man. Research institutions, the Menninger Foundation and Edger Cayce's A.R.E. Clinic in Virginia Beach, Virginia, have documented his spiritual healings. Krippner and Villoldo also led an international group to South America to witness spiritual healing and experience shamanic initiation, which they reported in their 1986 book *Healing States*.

When Krippner asked his teacher, don Eduardo, to initiate members of this tour group, the Peruvian shaman agreed, because he was told in a vision to share his healing and shamanism knowledge with outsiders. The spirit world is directing its mediators, the modern shamans, to teach today's citizens to be stewards of the earth.

How Does Shamanism Work?

The word *shaman* comes from a Siberian tribal language, describing a woman or man who enters an altered state of consciousness to journey into other realms of reality. Castaneda calls these other worlds "nonordinary reality." Harner coined the term "shamanic state of consciousness" (SCC). This altered state is induced by drumming, chanting, or taking natural hallucinogens. Neo-shamanism adds flotation tanks, active-alert hypnosis, strobe lights, and mind-altering machines to the list of SSC inducers.

Shamans can move between ordinary and extraordinary reality at will. They make the journeys to spirit realms to bring balance between the dark and the light, the Upper, Middle, and Lower worlds. Shamans believe people, especially modern folks, are caught in a cultural trance that limits the possibilities of their universe. Changing perceptions of reality can influence real world events such as the progress of disease and the improvement of health. The shamans' role is to bring back information to their clients and community to help alter the perceptions and experience of an illness. It can be a dangerous journey.

There are many kinds of spirits or energies, good and bad, in the reality beyond ours. Shamans, the "wounded healers" of their societies, have usually overcome personal pain or injury. Suffering develops the courage and fortitude needed for the trip to those other worlds.

This journey distinguishes shamans from psychic healers. Generally, spirits possess psychics and illnesses are taken on by faith healers. Shamans, on the other hand, travel out to their guides, into the spirit realms, to do their healing work.

Shamans call on guardian spirits and power animals to protect and guide them and supply them with special, personal power. European tradition called these spirits "companions" or "familiars." Traditionally, witches worked their magic through familiars such as black cats.

Power animals represent knowledge and power, the elemental energy of nature. They are very real to the shaman, an alter ego. We all have guardian spirits. The difference is that the shaman can actively use the power from these entities at will, tapping into that power and entering a shamanic state of consciousness for specific reasons and needs.

Shamans employ many different tools and techniques to connect themselves, and their charges, with the spiritual. The use of hallucinogens is a common induction method. Taking peyote is a sacred rite. A Ladakh lama-shaman rings a bell to bring up the life force of his patient. Sweat lodges, skin- or blanket-covered huts heated by hot rocks in the center, cleanse the body and clear the minds of troubled tribal members.

A shaman will lay out power objects on a mesa (table or high plateau). Each piece embodies the power it symbolizes. While many symbols vary from culture to culture, medicine men and women use the altar for sorting out and influencing the forces of nature to diagnose and heal disease.

Many of these ritual tools and techniques are being adapted and refined for contemporary society. Dr. Lewis Mehl integrates his medical training with shamanic ritual, prayers, and stories from his Cherokee and Lakota heritage. Co-author of the book *Pregnancy as Healing,* Mehl also specializes in obstetrics. His complementary medicine practice includes visualization, somatic therapy, body awareness training, and biofeedback to support women with high-risk pregnancies.

Dr. Mehl treats patients with ailments such as asthma, Epstein-Barr syndrome, cancer, and uterine fibroids, as well. His seminars on treating chronic conditions are laced with examples of tribal traditions and explanations of how he uses them with patients. Mehl's approach highlights the psychology of shamanic medicine, an important factor in all healings.

Neo-shamanic psychology is empowering individuals to discover their own connections to the spirit and create their own healing rituals and tools. Harner Method shamanic counseling uses the unique tactic of inducing clients into a shamanic state of consciousness by listening, via headphones, to taped ritual drumming. The client narrates aloud her own journey into the spirit realm, while the counselor coaches and listens. The session is taped for later therapeutic discussion and analysis. Clients learn to make contact with their power animals, getting answers for themselves from wise ones or guardian spirits.

Attendance at seminars and classes in Shamanism is rising. Some groups meet monthly to learn about medicine wheel circles, prayer sticks, imagery, and guided visualization in various shamanic traditions. It is a modern initiation schedule to fit today's busy lifestyles. While many use these experiences for personal spiritual transformation and self-healing, all these classes, books, tours, and gatherings are fueling the global healing movement.

The very essence of native spiritualism is our place *in* nature, not over it. It's an entirely different attitude than the philosophy of Judeo-Christian culture. Students learn about tribal animism, the belief that all things are alive, and Native American reverence for the Earth. They grow to recognize their profound connection to nature. This sensitizes adherents to the fragile condition of Earth's life-support systems, turning some into newborn environmentalists.

What Happens in a Shamanism Course?

Anthropologist Angeles Arrien teaches a shamanism course from her cross-cultural perspective. Students sit in the medicine wheel, learning to celebrate the year with typical seasonal rituals. Winter is a time of gestation and incubation, an opportunity to focus on "cave work," or inner processing. Spring is the time of the visionary. The new native comes out of the cave to sing, tell stories, and plant seeds. Summer is the healer's season, a time to open oneself to the abundance of life. Fall is for completion and closure; rituals focus on the power of silence and gathering the harvest.

In this particular group, Arrien leads her students on a vision quest weekend during each of the three "outer" seasons—spring, summer, and fall (winter is "cave time"). Vision quests are times to commune with nature and spirit, to spend time in silence, and to work on oneself and the theme of the season.

Other shamanic gatherings may build sweat lodges. Or participants fast, pray, and speak in spirit tongues (without blame or judgment) to cleanse and heal both body and mind. There are a growing number of sacred shamanic activities, offered from a variety of sources that can be used in healing our modern lives.

Cautions for Exploring Shamanism

In tribal societies, community members know their shaman. Their healer has suffered the transformative wound or gone through initiation among the people she or he will serve. In our mobile society, however, we have no mechanism to sort out the sorcerer from the sincere. More and more publications and events help curious persons explore neo-shamanism. With no national organization or professional certification program to make the process easy, individuals must check out their potential teachers or activities themselves.

It is important to ask questions about the manner and length of apprenticeship. Talk to former and current students of the seminar leader or medicine person. Listen and evaluate what you hear. Check your gut feelings to see if what you hear and are asked to do feels right for you.

Whether you believe in the Native spirit world or not, tragedies like Jonestown show us that the human mind can fall under the spell of dangerous powers. We need to care for our own spirit and self with the same reverence with which our Native American guides hold all life.

READ MORE ABOUT IT

SHAMANISM

The Way of the Shaman
by Michael Harner
(New York: Bantam Books, 1980)

Shamanism: Archaic Techniques of Ecstasy
by Mircea Eliade
(Princeton: Princeton University Press, 1964)

Shamanism: An Expanded View of Reality
edited by Shirley Nicholson
(Wheaton, IL: Theosophical Publishing House, 1987)

Medicine Woman
by Lynn Andrews
(New York: Harper & Row, 1981)

Imagery in Healing: Shamanism and Modern Medicine
by Jean Achterberg
(Boston: Shambala, 1985)

Shamanic Voices: A Survey of Visionary Narratives
by Joan Halifax
(New York: E. P. Dutton, 1979)

*Healing States: Journey Into The World of Spiritual Healing &
    Shamanism*
by Alberto Villoldo and Stanley Krippner
(New York: Simon & Schuster, 1986)

RESOURCES

The Foundation for Shamanic Studies
P.O. Box 670, Belden Station
Norwalk, CT 06852
(203) 454-2827
❏ information
❏ workshops
❏ membership
❏ research
❏ training and certification

Dance of the Deer Foundation
P.O. Box 699
Soquel, CA 95073
(408) 475-9560
❏ information
❏ training

T'ai Chi, Aikido, and Other Martial Arts

 ### *What Is a Martial Art?*

Martial arts are systems of physical and mental training used for self-understanding, expression through movement, and self-defense. Primarily Asian practices, they are also found in other parts of the world, such as South America. Martial arts evolved out of ritual dances and various forms of combat—hand-to-hand, sword, spear or staff.

The most popular philosophies and techniques were developed in China and Japan. The marital arts most available in the U.S. include:

❏ *Aikido* (Japanese)

❏ *Chi Gung* or *Qi Gong* (Chinese)

❏ *Judo* (Japanese)

❏ *Jujitsu* (Japanese)

❏ *Karate* (Japanese)

❏ *Kendo* (Japanese)

❏ *Kung Fu* (Chinese)

❏ *Tae Kwon Do* (Korean)

❏ *T'ai Chi Ch'uan* (Chinese)

Today, individuals adopt them as part of a spiritual quest, for self-defense, and as a lifestyle health practice. Some advanced forms of martial arts train their students in healing techniques, channeling the life energy forces of *chi*, or *ki*.

History and Development of the Martial Arts

The roots of many martial arts reach back to ancient ritual dances. More than 5,000 years ago, the Chinese celebrated a festival called *No*. Twelve participants danced through the streets portraying the animals of the Chinese zodiac. Led by a shaman (tribal priest-healer) in a bear mask, the ceremonial dance purified the village before the New Year.

Dances celebrated folk heroes and nature as well as animals, and the particular dance movements became the bases for yoga-like exercises. These were finally systematized into a health practice by a first-century Taoist physician. They began to be used to balance organs, to relieve leg cramps from long hours of sitting meditation, and to relax the body. As barbarians invaded the country, monks learned to speed up the motions and convert the passive exercises into aggressive self-defense techniques. For example, they could use the hitherto benign "Ape Steals Fruit" gesture to pluck out an opponent's eye. The martial arts were also used in the rivalries between religious sects and in champion contests waged between feudal armies to decide a battle.

The myths about historical origins vary for different Chinese martial arts. *Kung Fu,* kicked into the minds and hearts of Americans by David Carradine's hit television show of the '70s, actually originated in the Shao Lin monastery. The Indian Buddhist monk, Budhidharma, who brought Zen to China in the fifth century, taught these Honan province monks a boxing method that eventually developed into the 170 movements practiced in kung fu today.

There are four stories explaining the creation of T'ai Chi. But the most popular myth is that the Taoist monk, Chang Sanfeng, invented the movements after dreaming about a strange fight-dance between a snake and bird. In Tao, the bird commonly symbolizes universal consciousness; the snake, earthbound consciousness or the regenerative powers of nature. Whatever their origins, his first 13 movements eventually grew into the present 108 relaxed postures. Practiced by flowing from one pose into the other without a break, t'ai chi expresses the blending of the eternal and temporal, heaven and earth.

T'ai Chi Ch'uan, meaning Supreme Ultimate Power and sometimes called *Ch'ang Ch'uan* (Long Boxing), enjoyed a fad status in the 1850s in China. When Chairman Mao came to power in 1949, he advocated t'ai chi ch'uan as a health practice, a means to eliminate stress-related diseases.

In 1956, the government standardized t'ai chi exercises, creating a simplified version of just 24 movements. You may remember seeing news pictures during Nixon's historic 1972 trip that showed early morning streets lined with old and young citizens doing this moving meditation. They were most likely practicing the government-approved version.

In Japan, *budo* is the generic term for martial arts. As in China, each martial art is part of a philosophical discipline, a path or *do*. Each form has its own highly developed teaching tradition and philosophy. *Karate,* whose name means "Chinese Hands," grew out of kung fu. *Jujitsu* and its derivative, *judo,* also show influence of Chinese forms of wrestling and grappling. Sports developed for the samurai military class during the peaceful Edo period (1600s and 1700s), these martial arts were used to redirect warriors' fighting spirit and energy.

Founded by Dr. Jigoro Kano in the late 1800s, Kodokan College in Tokyo regulates and establishes the rules for judo throughout the world. This learned man worked hard to emphasize the discipline and philosophy of judo, as well as the modified holds, strikes, and throws, as he promoted it throughout the world. Today judo, which means "the gentle way," is recognized as a competition sport in the U.S. and at the Olympics.

Aikido is a modern development. Founded in the 1920s by a Japanese farmer and martial arts expert, Morihei Uyeshiba, its name means the "Way of Spiritual Harmony." Morihei studied many of the traditional Japanese martial arts, mastering skills with the sword, staff, and spear, as well as judo and jujitsu style techniques. One form he mastered was a composite system, *"Daito-ryu Aiki-jutsu."* (The term *aiki* means to unite or harmonize [*ai*] life energy or vital force [*ki*].) Morihei also pursued spiritual practices in the Shinto and Buddhist traditions.

One spring day in 1925, while sitting in his garden, Morihei received a divine inspiration that the true purpose of budo was love, love that cherishes and nourishes all beings. He began to teach his own method. Morihei's skills, particularly in anticipating blows and handling several attackers at a time, won him many followers. In a ten-year period during and after World War II, Morihei consolidated his techniques and perfected the religious philosophy into what he now called "aikido," making it a true spiritual discipline.

In 1948, the "Aikikai," or Aiki Association was founded and began promoting Aikido in Japan and abroad. Morihei gained world recognition as "O-Sensei," the master of Aikido, and received several decorations from the Japanese government. He died in 1969, instructing his disciples: "Aikido is for the entire world. Train not for selfish reasons, but for all people everywhere."

How Do the Martial Arts Work?

Training in the martial arts can be healthy for the mind, body, and spirit. Choose one that fits your personality, health needs, and values or philosophical orientation.

Karate, judo, and other competition-based forms are vigorous self-defense and strengthening exercises. T'ai chi, the most gentle and individual of the arts, is a form of meditation while in motion. It has gained the respect of medical personnel for its ability to tone the body without strain. Aikido, based on cooperation and the give-and-take of a two-person relationship, is always done with partners.

A form of the Philippine martial art, *arnis,* called *sinewali,* uses one or two long staff rods. Students at JFK University practice an adaptation by Stuart Heller called "Sticks," for stress response training. Opponents hit each other's sticks in prescribed patterns to gain awareness of how various emotional reactions to these mini-shocks affect their bodies, minds and movements.

A 400-year-old Brazilian art form, *capoeira,* mixes acrobatics and dance. It is a form of both exercise and self-defense, and can be an aerobic practice. The only indigenous American martial art, *capoeira* was developed by the African slaves in Brazil.

In China, martial arts are divided into two types. *Wai chia,* or "outer family" arts, are Buddhist-inspired and originate from outside China, usually India. They emphasize muscular strength, conditioning, and endurance. Kung fu is an outer family art; judo and karate are Japanese equivalents. These forms consist of static postures and hard, linear movements, kicks, and punches. Kung fu kicks stretch the joints and ligaments. With long-term practice, they can gradually loosen the hamstrings, allowing full rotation of the femur. Kung fu can be aerobic as well. An hour standing in a low "horse stance" (knees bent), punching out the right and left fists alternately, can provide the same workout as an hour of jogging.

Some studies show that Eastern "combat sports" can curb violent tendencies. Western athletics focus on skills and physical strength, and only recently have begun to recognize the role of the mind in optimum performance. The martial arts, however, require a blending of mind and body. Full fighting force is achieved by focusing energy, controlling the emotions, and overcoming aggression. The ritualistic nature and philosophy of the martial arts teach strict rules of conduct and respect for one's opponent.

The other branch of Chinese martial arts is the *nei chai* or "inner family." Taoist-inspired and developed within China, these forms aim to cultivate vital energy and economy of strength. Movements are slow and fluid, performed meditatively. T'ai chi is a typical example. Other nei chai include *Pa Kua Chang,* a coiling, spiraling exercise, and *Hsing I Ch'uan,* a linear, spirited series of rising and falling gestures. The t'ai chi philosophy looks to the I Ching and involves Taoist meditation. It also includes a sensitivity exercise, called "sticking," in which participants mirror the movement of a partner.

Done slowly, these arts can build health and cultivate peace of mind. Performed rapidly, the gestures can unleash devastating blows for self-defense. In fact, t'ai chi also has a free-style sparring form with special weapons. However, popular emphasis is on its meditative qualities and philosophical wisdom.

Nei chai arts emphasize the principles of relaxing and sinking, which both build energy and reduce tension. Relaxing means maintaining constant yet light muscle tension while using the minimum effort necessary for any movement. The muscles work in a continual yielding-and-advancing rhythm. This promotes muscle toning without stress or strain. A University of Toronto study confirms that t'ai chi increases body flexibility.

Sinking involves simultaneously dropping weight through the feet, trusting the support of the ground, and releasing any tension in the belly. This allows fuller breathing, which promotes body lightness. It also "roots" energy for a grounding effect. This kind of nonexertion counterbalances our Western cultural training to strive and work hard at "doing" an exercise.

T'ai Chi can be moderate exercise, raising oxygen consump-

294 The Encyclopedia of Alternative Health Care

tion 40 to 50 percent. It can raise one's heart rate as well—usually within a normal training target zone. The deeper and faster you do the postures, the more oxygen consumption increases and muscles strengthen.

Chinese doctors often prescribe t'ai chi as complementary treatment for many conditions. Particularly suited as a health practice for the weak, elderly, and infirm, it improves blood and lymph circulation. Increased energy flow also helps ward off illness and fatigue.

Like t'ai chi, aikido stresses "non-doing," letting the body act in a smooth and natural way that reduces habitual tension. Both use fluid and circular movements and emphasize personal development and awareness or sensitivity. And both treat the mind and body as one.

However, aikido is practiced with a partner. Devoid of competition, the focus is on harmonizing with the partner's movements, rather than fighting an opponent. The throws and falls of aikido teach how to work with the partner's energy flow and then how to redirect it. However, the partner's safety is a primary responsibility; the object is to throw without harming the other.

Aikido is a way to reframe combat aggression into peacefulness. Aikido focuses awareness on the lower abdomen, the *hara,* one's emotional and physical center. To develop hara is to cultivate maturity, empathy, and calmness. The goal is to attain balance and centering, to be alert, at rest, and poised to move in any direction at any moment.

What Happens in Martial Arts Classes?

The traditional form of t'ai chi has 128 postures, including repetitions, and takes 15–20 minutes at a proper (slow) speed. Some teachers create their own short forms, anywhere from 35 to 50 poses, cutting the repeated positions. The short forms may take from seven to ten minutes. Some traditionalists turn up their noses at these superficial "fast-food" versions. However, they are easy to adopt as daily routines, to do upon rising in the morning or just before bed.

There are many books on the various styles of t'ai chi. However, it is essential to start with a real live teacher. T'ai chi movements are too subtle and complex to learn without an observer and coach to encourage and correct your first efforts.

Even while learning t'ai chi in a class, practice is most often a solitary task. Each person must find his own rhythm and flow. If you've seen pictures of people on the streets of Peking performing their morning exercises, you probably noticed that they looked as if they were in their own world. That is the meditative nature of t'ai chi.

And remember, t'ai chi and the martial arts are not just exercise routines. Serious students must commit to long-term study, not simply of the postures but also of the philosophy. T'ai chi devotees delve into the I Ching, Taoism, and often other kinds of meditation and spiritual persuits.

Aikido, on the other hand, can't be done alone. Morihei's purpose was to create a form that promotes respect for and bonding with others. Classes of up to 30 people work out in a special practice room, called a *dojo*. Sessions cater to various levels of proficiency. Strict decorum must be maintained, even if you are just observing a class. At my first visit, I was reprimanded for crossing my arms while I watched.

Class starts with a brief meditation and with limbering exercises. In advanced classes, the warm-up looks like a basketball drill, except each participant is running to make a fall rather than to do a lay-up.

The meat of each class is learning new throws or holding mechanisms. The focus is on the technique, not whether you manage to throw somebody. It is a breach of form, for instance, to throw someone so that any part of her body lands off the edge of the mat. That was one of my early mistakes. I wanted to "win" by always being the thrower, never the throwee. The teacher stopped the class, using me to make a point. I found out the importance of maintaining proper form and learned to drop my goal-directedness.

In fact, the first lesson was learning how to fall: rolling on my shoulder and up onto my feet again, ready for the next action. I finally perceived the grace in being thrown, a result of blending energies with my partner. And the lesson has come in handy in everyday life. Now when I roller-skate and jam my wheel on a stick or stone, I save my wrists and knees by offering the ground my shoulder and rolling with the fall, rather than bracing against it.

Competitive martial arts, such as judo, require rigorous training. Practiced in a dojo or gymnasium, students learn perfect posture and balance in order to do the kicks and throws. The devotee's ability to use good judgment, make quick decisions under pressure, and perform the various kicks, holds, and throws wins a match. The goal is to immobilize the opponent in a certain position for a certain time or force her to give up by using special strangleholds or arm locks.

These wrestling techniques have also been adapted for self-defense. Women across the country are taking classes at continuing education centers, health clubs, and schools to learn how to neutralize, overcome, and/or escape attackers. Not only does proficiency arm you for the streets, but it also builds self-confidence and self-trust. I think it is one of the best gifts a woman can give herself.

Applications and Cautions

The list of benefits of consistent and long-term practice of t'ai chi is long. It ranges from improving muscle tone and physiological self-regulation to cultivating poise and a tranquil spirit.

T'ai chi's gentle leg-raising movements massage and strengthen the intestines, aiding waste elimination. The slow, soft turning and bending motions massage other organs. T'ai chi calms both body and mind, its meditative quality relieving stress and anxiety. This provides effective cotreatment for ulcers and other nervous disorders.

T'ai chi deepens breathing, increasing oxygen to the blood, which opens blood vessels and allows the heart to function more smoothly. It also opens joints, especially the knees, alleviating inflammatory diseases such as arthritis and rheumatism, and strengthens the lower back.

The martial arts promote improved balance, physical coordination, agility, and stamina. Reflexes and instinctual behavior sharpen, as can concentration and memory. Relief from pain, stress, and muscular tensions leads to more precise nervous control over bodily functions and refined movements.

The focus on cultivating *chi* or *ki* builds a reserve of vital force. The positive results might include enhanced sexual functioning and increased psychic energy. In fact, both the Chinese and Japanese martial arts traditions include vital energy healing techniques. The same life force used to attack or defend can be channeled to heal. Students learn to direct energy from their bodies out through their hands, targeting an injured or dysfunctional part of their own, or another body.

I have experienced *chi* healing energy. A *chi kung* master visiting JFK University tried to explain to me how his martial arts practice opened energy meridians and strengthened organ functions. Struggling with his heavily accented English, he finally just showed me how he could send the *chi* energy. He placed his hands over my palms, and I immediately felt a vibrating warmth flow up my arms to my face.

Chi kung can be a static practice, focusing only on internal energy flow. Iron Shirt Chi Kung strengthens or energizes fasciae (connective tissues), tendons, and bone structure and marrow (for blood building). Used to help the debilitated build *chi,* it's suitable for chemotherapy patients.

Before undertaking any martial arts exercise program, it is important to consult your primary care provider. Remember that the "outer" martial arts, such as karate, kung fu, and judo, require sharp kicks and the ability to sustain the impact of blows and falls. Aikido involves throws and rolling on the mat. People with serious mechanical disorders, back pain, or recent injuries should get an OK from primary care providers before starting any training or classes.

The benefits of practicing a martial art can reach beyond physical well-being. Philosophical insights gained through my aikido classes began to help in my marketing management work. Remember that Morihei would take on several opponents or partners at a time, anticipating each one's plan of attack. He was ready to move in any direction at any moment. I began to perceive myself as poised at my desk like an aikido master at the center of the mat. I translated that readiness to my job, becoming better able to respond to the many unexpected and sometimes demoralizing pressures of work.

READ MORE ABOUT IT

T'AI CHI AND OTHER MARTIAL ARTS

Cheng Tzu's Thirteen Treatises on T'ai Chi Ch'uan
by Man-chi'ing Cheng
(Berkeley: North Atlantic Books, 1985)

The Tao of Tai Chi Chuan
by Tsung Hwa Jou
(Rutland, VT: Charles E. Tuttle, 1980)

Chinese Healing Arts: Internal Kung Fu
edited by William R. Berk
(Burbank, CA: Unique Publications, 1986)

Iron Shirt Chi Kung
by Mantak Chai
(Huntington, NY: Healing Tao Books, 1986)

Aikido and the New Warrior
by Richard Strozzi Heckler
(Berkeley: North Atlantic Books, 1985)

Aikido
by Kisshomara Uyeshiba
(Tokyo: Hozanshi Publishing, 1974)

Judo: the Gentle Way
Alan Fromm and Nicolas Soames
(London: Routledge and Kegan Paul, 1982)

RESOURCES

Healing Tao Center
P.O. Box 1194
Huntington, NY 11743
(516) 549-9452
❏ publications
❏ products
❏ retreats
❏ workshops (nationwide)

The School of T'ai Chi Ch'uan, Inc.
47 West 13th Street, 5th floor
New York, NY 10011
(212) 929-1981
❏ information
❏ trainings and classes (also Chicago, Florida)

Zen-Do Kai Martial Arts Association
12 West Main Street
P.O. Box 186
Johnstown, NY 12005
(518) 762-4723
❏ information
❏ newsletter
❏ classes

U.S. Aikido Federation
Central Headquarters
98 State Street
Northampton, MA 01060
(413) 586-7122
❏ club lists
❏ seminars
❏ trainings

Therapeutic Touch

 ### What Is Therapeutic Touch?

Therapeutic Touch (TT) is a laying-on of hands healing technique created by a professor of nursing for other health care professionals to use to enhance patient care and treatment progress. Inspired by research on the effectiveness of psychic healing, it is based on human energy transfer in the act of healing. However, TT is designed to be done by the nonpsychic who has a strong intent to help or heal recipients.

History and Development of Therapeutic Touch

While most cultures dating back to the caves of ancient Europe have a tradition of hands-on healing, laying-on of hands has somehow gotten lost among the high technology and scientific precision of modern medicine. It took a nursing teacher to translate common wisdom from traditional medicines into a form acceptable to modern medical personnel. Dolores Krieger was a new Ph.D. in Nursing and teaching at New York University when she joined a research team in nearby upstate New York in 1971. Otelia Bengssten, M.D. and Dora Kuntz, a clairvoyant and healer herself, wanted to study the effect of direct laying-on of hands treatment by a well-known Hungarian healer, Oscar Estebany. Krieger joined the team as a health care professional and chose a biochemical measure for healer energy influence—blood hemoglobin levels—in the study's 19 medically-referred subjects.

Krieger knew of Bernard Grad's experiments with Estebany at McGill University in Canada. Results showed a significant increase in chlorophyll in plants and accelerated wound healing in mice. Krieger reasoned that hemoglobin's biochemical makeup and role in humans was similar to chlorophyll's structure and function in plant life. Hemoglobin is integral to many life-sustain-

300

ing functions in the body, including transporting oxygen from the lungs to cellular tissue and removing toxins from the body via the liver. Positive effects on hemoglobin would enhance the body's healing ability.

The experiment, in which Estebany both touched the patients and also briefly held "magnetically charged" cotton batting to leave with the subjects, showed elevated blood levels of hemoglobin. Krieger was also surprised by reports of improvement of or relief from symptoms by a majority of the participants. Their diagnoses had ranged from rheumatoid arthritis and emphysema to pancreatitis and brain tumor. Krieger wondered whether the healing touch could only be done by someone born with a gift for healing.

Krieger decided to study with Kunz to see if she, Krieger, a nonpsychic with no natural "healing" ability (that she knew of) could learn to do what Estebany did in the experiment. Krieger discovered that not only did she feel the energy flow and thus affect people, but also that the more she did it, the easier and better she got at it.

With the help of Dora Kunz, she created a technique to teach to other health care professionals. Knowing that anything that smacked of psychic healing would alienate most people in her medical world, Krieger decided to call it "Therapeutic Touch," a simple name that says what it really is.

Krieger started teaching Therapeutic Touch in 1975 in a class at NYU called "Frontiers in Nursing." Soon nursing students took their new-found skills into private and public hosptials, using it on patients who agreed to try "a little experiment." Her students came back with more and more testimonials to TT's positive effects.

Krieger wrote *The Therapeutic Touch: How to Use Your Hands to Help and Heal* in 1979. The book is a simple step-by-step explanation of how to learn to do TT. It also includes early scientific studies as well as many of the interesting experiences both Krieger and some of her students have had with Therapeutic Touch. In 1987, Krieger published *Living the Therapeutic Touch: Healing As a Lifestyle,* which reveals more of her personal experiences with TT, demonstrating the profound philosophical effect it can have on one's life.

Krieger and her students have shared TT with thousands of health care professionals throughout the U.S. and in 38 countries, teaching the technique at universities, in hospital in-service programs, and continuing education courses.

How Does Therapeutic Touch Work?

Krieger sees the therapeutic use of hands as a universal human act, a gift we've forgotten in our scientific, mechanistic, "synthetic and frequently anti-human" era. Her research into the healing touch led her to note that, throughout history, from cave drawings in the Pyrenees (estimated to be 15,000 years old) and stories in the Bible, to historical figures such as the Norwegian king Olaf and the kings of France and England, people practiced laying-on of hands to heal. She wanted to know why touch is therapeutic. Her conclusion: touch can transfer energy.

Besides her background in nursing and neurophysiology, Krieger had studied the health practices of yoga and Ayurvedic medicine, as well as Tibetan and Chinese medicine. She connects the Hindu and yogic concept of *prana*, or life energy, to the rise in blood levels of hemoglobin and its bioenergetic and physiological effects in healing. The Hindus believe that *prana* is a subtle energetic component of sunlight taken in from the environment to the body via the breath. Hemoglobin transports oxygen from the air in the lungs to all parts of the body, fueling our bodies' life-sustaining functions.

Healers and healthy people have an abundance of *prana;* sick people have a relative deficiency of *prana.* Krieger sees Therapeutic Touch as making a connection, like jumper cables, between the healer's charged battery and the sick person's low battery. The sick one borrows energy to get his immune system jump-started and energized to handle whatever disease or condition is distressing him.

Increased hemoglobin is only one indication of the therapeutic effects of touch. Further research by Krieger and other nurses demonstrated that TT induces a state of physiological relaxation, reduces anxiety, and is effective in reducing postoperative pain and relieving headaches. One of the most moving stories in *Therapeutic Touch* is of a nursing student who gave birth to a premature baby so early that its chance of survival was in question. Krieger gave quick lessons on TT to the mother, who then applied it to her baby, resulting in dramatic weight gain and neurological progress. Staff and some of the parents of other "preemies" asked this nurse to teach them what she did for her child. TT became a standard practice in that hospital's premature infant unit—and in other hospitals as well.

Janet Quinn, Ph.D., R.N., one of Krieger's first students and an associate professor at the Unviersity of South Carolina's College of Nursing, found that actual contact between the healer and the ailing was not necessary. Moving the hands just above a patient's body can sometimes transfer energy more effectively than direct touch. She points out the role of impersonal or unconditional love in the healing—a message mystics and metaphysical literature have laid out for centuries.

Dolores Krieger has brought to bear the rigor and power of modern science, insisting on and supporting documented research on her technique, a simple mode of healing based on ancient wisdom. And, whether one believes in *prana* or unconditional love, the fact is that this technique can be done without any belief in psychic healing or background in ancient Oriental medicine. It only requires a relatively healthy body and the intent to help or heal.

What Happens in a Session?

A patient or receiver can be sitting or lying, conscious or unconscious, to receive Therapeutic Touch. The healer or nurse usually asks permission to give a hands-on session. Before touching the patient, however, she centers herself in a meditative state, focusing on her intent to help or heal the individual. This is a crucial step. In the research on TT, nurses who did not center themselves or focus healing intent but concentrated on counting backward in increments of seven while going through the hand motions of a TT session showed no significant effects on their patients. The meditative state and focused intent are vital parts of TT.

The next steps of TT are to assess the patient's energy field and then transmit energy as appropriate. Classes or self-training in TT help the healer sensitize her hands to pressure, magnetic feelings and/or temperature changes under her hands that indicate an energy block or distressed area of the body. Signals from the hands help her assess imbalances in the patient's energy field or the energy surrounding and penetrating the body. As Krieger and her students point out, experience and practice are the best teachers.

The Therapeutic Touch healer perceives energy as being congested, similar to acupuncture's concept of blocked energy in the meridians. The first hand motions are to "unruffle the field." A ruffled field can feel dense or lethargic. Sweeping away heat or pressure begins the energy flow, preparing the way for the actual healing act. I have felt the pressure of a headache around my head almost "pop" when my field is unruffled, the tension beginning to drain out as my friend makes long, purposeful sweeps around my head and down my neck and back.

The heart of TT is the directing and modulating of energy. Hands assess the imbalances of energy in various parts of the patient's energy field and then begin to move that energy around. The patient may need energy moved from one part to another, from congested stomach area to deficient lower limbs, for example.

If the patient is quite ill or weak, the healer will transfer energy from herself to her patient. This is why one must be relatively healthy to do Therapeutic Touch. The healer's energy battery must be charged so as not to deplete itself. Energy transference feels like radiating warmth or heat to me.

My first experience with Therapeutic Touch was when I had just come out of a three-hour operation and I felt like a Mack truck had parked on my chest. I could barely raise myself beyond the ground fog of postoperative pain and the effects of anaesthetics. My friend Sue Ann massaged my feet and then applied TT to the site of my operation. First I felt the pressure release and then I perceived radiating warmth and caring infusing my aching body. I left the hospital a day earlier than expected.

The healer can sense when the energy field feels balanced and when to stop TT. Often the receiver will look refreshed, his face flushed with hemoglobin-rich blood, or even be in a deep state of relaxation. The waves of pain or the anxiety attack have subsided, the tension or discomfort relieved. The healer may assess with her hands to see whether more Therapeutic Touch is required. She usually finishes by shaking her hands or running cold water over them to clear any excess charge.

Applications and Cautions

TT can be used alongside any treatment program for conditions from postoperative pain to acute or chronic illness. Contraindications are for diseases such as cancer, where increased energy flow, metabolism, or circulation could encourage the spread of the pathology.

READ MORE ABOUT IT

THERAPEUTIC TOUCH

Therapeutic Touch: How to Use Your Hands to Heal
by Dolores Krieger, Ph.D., R.N.
(Englewood Cliffs, NJ: Prentice Hall, 1979)

Therapeutic Touch: A Practical Guide
by Janet Macrae
(Westminster, MD: Alfred A. Knopf, 1987)

Therapeutic Touch
edited by Marianne Borelli and Patricia Holt
(New York: Springer Publishing, 1986)

RESOURCES

Nurse Healers—Professional Association, Inc.
175 Fifth Avenue, Suite 3399
New York, New York 10010
❑ referrals
❑ information

Tragerwork

What Is Trager Psychophysical Integration?

The Trager Approach, also commonly called Tragerwork or Tragering, is an intuitive method of body-mind work created by a boxer and acrobat turned M.D. Milton Trager's combination of hands-on and movement techniques is practiced in a relaxed meditative state, called *hook-up*.

Practitioners use light, gentle, nonintrusive hand and mind movements to break up and release deep-seated physical and mental patterns that restrict the muscles' range of motion. The aim is to remind the individual of what it feels like to feel good again.

History and Development of Tragerwork

In 1926, Milton Trager was an 18-year-old professional boxer in Miami. A trainer remarked on Trager's skill at giving a rubdown, making Trager realize he had a gift in his hands. After successfully working on his father's sciatica and on the complaints of a few other neighbors, he quit boxing to save his hands and became instead an acrobat and dancer.

One day Trager was working out on the beach with his brother, when he decided to try jumping *softer* instead of higher. This opened a new world to explore: how to perform movements in an effortless manner.

Trager was drawn deeper and deeper into the study of physical health and by 1941 completed a Doctorate of Physical Medicine at the L.A. College of Drugless Physicians. Certified in California to practice in the field of neuromuscular disorders, he specialized in treating polio patients.

Eight years later, at age 41, Trager decided he wanted to become a doctor, but was rejected by 70 U.S. medical schools.

The University Autonome de Guadalajara in Mexico did take him. And, after he demonstrated his bodywork technique on a patient, the medical school opened a polio rehabilitation clinic which Trager ran while he earned his M.D. degree.

After graduating, Trager moved to Hawaii and opened a private medical practice. For almost 20 years, he kept a low profile, working on some of his patients and perfecting his neuromuscular technique. Like many pioneers in the new health care revolution, Trager was "discovered" after he demonstrated at Esalen, the center for the human potential movement, in 1975. His success with difficult neuromuscular disorders, such as multiple sclerosis and accident trauma, inspired one satisfied client, Betty Fuller, to propose the creation of an institute to teach Trager's work.

The Trager Institute was organized in 1977. A few years later, Trager closed his practice in Hawaii to devote himself full time to the training and certification of Trager workers. By the late 1980s, there were more than 1,000 practitioners and students in 18 countries.

Like Ida Rolf, Judith Aston, and other ground-breaking thinkers in bodywork therapies, Trager focused on developing and teaching his healing modality, not writing about it. He sometimes insists the method has no specific techniques, and relatively little has been published on it. *Trager Mentastics: Movement as a Way to Agelessness,* the first authorized book, came out in 1987. Meanwhile the Institute has put out only two journals in eight years. Like most intuitive arts, it must be experienced to really get a sense of it.

How Does the Trager Approach Work?

Tragerwork's aim is to break up neuromuscular holdings that often develop in response to accidents, illness, emotional trauma, poor movement and posture habits, as well as the everyday stresses of living. Tragerers see patterns of restrictive stiffness, tension, pain, and even functional limitations as products of an unconscious mental process. To illustrate, Trager tells the story of a surgery patient he observed.

Before surgery, the patient was so stiff that he had to turn his whole body to turn his head. Under anesthesia, the man was completely limp. Trager sat in the recovery room, watching the man's body become increasingly rigid as he came to, eventually returning to his original stiffness.

This incident convinced Trager that bodywork was strongly linked to mind work: that the body and mind are inseparable. The focus of his work became mind-to-mind communication between practitioner and client. The intention of Tragering is to allow the client to give up unconscious muscular control and sink into a deeply relaxed state.

The key to this communications is "hook-up," the ability of practitioners to perform their work in a relaxed, meditative state. Hook-up facilitates transmitting a sense of freedom, even playfulness, that is a fundamental part of the Tragering technique. It also heightens the practitioner's awareness of the client's tissue response (or lack of it). Is the mind getting the message to let go and let the body feel good?

The greatest benefit that Tragering can offer the client is a feeling that the body and mind are integrated and are able to work together to effect positive changes. These changes can be seen both in physical functioning and in other areas of the client's life.

Tragering can improve general physical functioning through releasing restricted and inhibited movement patterns, overlaying positive neuromuscular patterns at the source, the unconscious mind. Whether a polio client begins to walk again or an MS client gains better self-image just by feeling better, the improvements can change their lives.

What Happens in a Session?

The watchwords of a Trager session seem to be comfort, gentleness, and playfulness. Practitioners are careful to have a soothingly warm room and a well-padded table. Clients wear swimsuits or light, loose clothing; no oils or lotions are used. Sessions last from 1 to 1½ hours.

The practitioner's work is to create a safe, loving, nonjudgmental experience reminiscent of when we were babies cradled in our mothers' arms. The head, limbs, and trunk are rocked to invoke a freer, lighter feeling. Trager theorizes that rocking stimulates the cerebellum.

The Tragerer guides the client's passive body in a series of gentle, painless movements, making sure all the time that the client remains comfortable. The idea is to teach the body that it can feel good. Practitioners also use soft range-of-motion movements to test the limits of the client's mobility, and then gently rock the client past these limits.

Trager's theory is that given the choice between the old, painful, restrictive holdings and newer, freer, pleasurable movements, the unconscious mind will automatically choose freedom. That choice is communicated when the practitioner and the client achieve the hook-up. Trager people struggle for words to describe the experience, but the expressions on their faces during hook-up remind me of a meditative reverie—a state of peace, contentment, joy, release, and satisfaction.

Clients usually get Mentastics homework after each session. Mentastics is the active, self-guided version of the passive, individualized Trager session. Exercises are chosen to support progress made at each particular session. Tragerers are beginning to say that a good Mentastics workout can achieve as much as a session, or even more, because the client/exerciser is actively participating and learning to give himself good feelings.

I found the self-directed discovery intriguing. The leader would start us with "giving away our hand," having us push it up and out and then let it drop. Then she asked, how can we do it lighter? I had to pose this question in both mind and body, make the mental and physical connection to let go of my effort to do the move, and then let it just happen.

The lesson was about how, unconsciously, we expend unnecessary energy to do even the simplest movements. Absorbing this knowledge, I spotted other tense and wasteful expenditures of energy that I routinely made without ever before realizing it. I became aware, for example, of how I really bang on the computer keyboard when I work. Now I have found that if I let my fingers find their own, lighter touch, and release my clenched jaw as I work, writing becomes more playful for me. Trager would love it!

Applications and Cautions

Trager's particular specialty has been severe neuromuscular disturbances that do not respond well to conventional therapies. There are several stories of his successes with getting polio patients on their feet again. He has also worked with multiple sclerosis and muscular dystrophy, where Tragering's effects range from the experience of feeling better and enhancing self-image to increased mobility. However, some say that these effects are as much, or more, the results of Trager's innate healing energy, not his technique.

Trager practitioners work with a wide range of other debilitating conditions that limit movement, as well as with clients experiencing depression, poor posture, and everyday aches and pains. Tragerwork has also helped chronic back pain, migraine, high blood pressure, autism, emphysema, asthma, and sciatica. Tragerers continue to find their own applications of the technique.

Many athletes are finding Tragering helpful for their sports. Relaxation in movement is one of the keys to optimal performance, increasing stamina by encouraging suppleness and grace and conservation of energy in motion. Tennis players, for example, have found the added flexibility in both mind and body helps them handle the stress of competition. Tragering improves their ability to respond to the unexpected, and can facilitate more concentration and better emotional control. Golfers, cyclists, swimmers, runners, and body-builders are among the Trager enthusiasts.

The one area in which Trager advises caution is working with cancer and other autoimmune diseases. It is not so much that this gentle bodywork would do damage to such patients, but it is vital that they are being treated by other means. Also, while Tragerers will engage clients in dialogue about changes and issues in their lives as therapy continues, this counseling may not be sufficient. They refer people with significant psychoemotional conditions to psychotherapists.

READ MORE ABOUT IT

TRAGERWORK

Trager Mentastics: Movement as a Way to Agelessness
by Milton Trager, M.D.
(Barrytown, NY: Station Hill Press, 1987)

Job's Body: A Handbook for Bodywork
by Deane Juhan, M.A.
(Barrytown, NY: Station Hill Press, 1987)

RESOURCES

The Trager Institute
10 Old Mill Street
Mill Valley, CA 94941
(415) 388-2688
❑ trainings
❑ referrals
❑ workshops
❑ membership
❑ publications
❑ consultations

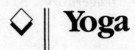

Yoga

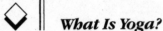

What Is Yoga?

Yoga is an ancient philosophical system and spiritual practice from India. Hindu texts define yoga as a means of deliverance from suffering, pain, and sorrow by mastering that which disturbs one's peace and harmony on the path to perfect union with God or the Universal Spirit. This union is reached through control of the mind, which must first overcome the distraction of fear and self-centeredness and unhealthy desires of the body and ego.

The yoga student's goal is to attain his or her highest possible degree of physical, mental, and spiritual integration to reach union. The practice includes various moving and static poses and stretches, breathing exercises, and diet and meditative disciplines meant to tone the mind, body, and soul.

History and Development of Yoga

The earliest evidence of yoga is the discovery of yoga positions engraved on seals from about 3000 B.C. Historians deduce that while poses, or *asanas,* were developed over time, the Indian sage Patanjali compiled the first textbook of yoga technique and wisdom from many ancient sources, perhaps about 250 B.C. *Yoga* is a Sanskrit word from the root *yui,* meaning to unite, bind, join or yoke. His *Yoga Sutras* is still the classic on yogic philosophy.

Through the centuries, yogis (people who follow the path of yoga) have demonstrated mastery of the body as well as freeing the mind and the spirit to experience cosmic union. In the 1920s, Western scientists came to India to test various yogi masters under laboratory conditions. These pioneers and other medical chroniclers who followed have recorded amazing physical feats

312

and powers. For example, some yogi's can slow or stop their breath and heartbeat for long periods, change blood pressure and body temperature, and control pain enough to lie on a bed of nails. These types of achievements inspired some of the early biofeedback research and development.

While yoga migrated west as a spiritual discipline, many people in the U.S. today explore yoga classes for their alternative style of exercise. Many *asanas* are valued for their gentle stretching action and low-impact workout. The modern American fitness era has also drawn interest to aerobic versions of yoga and yoga dance. Vegetarianism and non-violence are two more key elements of yoga philosophy that individuals and collective movements have adopted.

How Does Yoga Work?

Yoga practice focuses on a series of static or stretching exercises and breathing practices, as well as a meditation discipline and moral philosophy to reach a state of peace and harmony. In yoga, physical discipline is a means to an end—Samadhi, or a state of union with God.

On a physical level, yoga is a system for stress reduction. The science of yoga or yoga psychology sees that the most powerful source of stress is our mind. The effects of yoga poses, breathing exercises, meditation, and dietary disciplines on physiology help change poor mental and emotionlal habits that cause stress in our body.

Mental/emotional stress is a direct consequence of how we think of ourselves and relate to the world. For example, we see our boss frowning and think "She's displeased with me; I've done something wrong." Our reaction to this perception and interpretation is emotional; for example, fear of being berated or fired. Actually, that boss had too much for lunch and her stomach hurts; it has nothing to do with us. However, we can be conditioned by years of negative mental and emotional habits—i.e., assuming that we are wrong or feeling fear at the slightest negative-seeming sign—into a stress response.

Stress responses are our fight or flight mechanisms, originally designed to help us survive the dangers of primitive life, gone out of control in the relative ease of civilized, modern life.

They are out of control in the sense that we still experience the emotions and physiological reactions of being in danger when we get angry or frustrated with such civilized threats as freeway traffic and economic uncertainty.

The fight or flight syndrome releases adrenaline, changes respiration, and tenses muscle, stimulating us to respond to whatever we think threatens us. We normally discharge this high arousal state in the fight or flight that should follow. Unfortunately, flipping your lid over the car that just cut you off, or tossing and turning all night worrying about making the next mortgage payment isn't the same as wrestling a bear or running for your life. Your hormones are aroused but have no place to go.

Eventually, your body locks in as chronically aroused. We fall into a patterned reaction to almost everything. As babies, we naturally breathed from the belly (diaphragmatic breathing). But stressed by hunger or a wet bottom into crying, our chests would heave with each "waaaaa." As adults, we have learned to breathe from our upper chests, unless we are trained singers. Many women (and men) learn to hold in their stomachs to look slimmer, forcing breathing into the upper lungs. And all of us have tightened muscles somewhere—clenched jaws, stiff necks, rock-solid shoulders, or tense thighs. We weren't born that way. Those tensions are the results of chronic stress responses. Yoga can help change stress patterns.

Chest breathing is shallow and stimulates the right vagus nerve, a major regulator of autonomic functions such as heartbeat. Yoga breathing is belly breathing and stops stimulating the vagus, allowing it to do its job of keeping the heart rate in check. Yoga exercises stretch tensed muscles; coordinating breathing with movement increases the capacity of muscles to stretch. Diaphragmatic breathing expands lung space and enriches the blood with extra oxygen. This better nourishes the muscle tissue, which has more capacity to absorb the oxygen.

Meditation is one of the oldest relaxation techniques. Quieting the mind can quiet the body. The meditative state of yoga enhances our ability to observe physiological functions and their connections to emotional states and reactions. Developing an awareness and a sensitivity to what we feel and how these feelings express themselves in our bodies can lead to some measure of conscious control over many of these reactions. Consistent yoga practice in its whole—breath, asanas, diet, and mental discipline—can help you attain an attitude that helps you regulate the emotional and physiological states that contribute to stress and disease.

The Different Types of Yoga

If you choose to explore yoga as a health practice option, here are the different branches that have developed over time. Japanese scientist Hiroshi Motoyama identifies various yoga styles by primary focus or goal: spiritual, paranormal, and physiological. Some focus more on mental-spiritual activity than exercise. Others seem more body-oriented. They form a group that has been expanding from the original *Yoga Sutras* outline, as modern teachers continue to adapt the Indian wisdom and culture for the West.

Classical yoga identifies eight limbs or paths through actual practices which include: ethical (*yamas* and *hiyamas*), physical (*pranayamas* and *asanas*), mental, (*dharma*), and supramental (*dyyama*), and god-consciousness (*samadhi*). Some of the most common yoga practices or branches are:

❑ Bhakti is for those seeking the pathway to God through devotion and love.

❑ Jnana, the yoga of knowledge, has as its goal to attain *prajna,* or transcendental wisdom through meditation and thought; this is the yoga of the intellect.

❑ Karma is a yoga of service in action, emphasizing doing for others as a rememberance of God, and surrendering the rewards to God.

❑ Raja has as its object to realize directly the absolute self by stilling the mind through concentrated meditative effort (via *asanas* and *pranayama* breathing exercises) so the light of the internal spirit can shine through.

❑ Mantra or Nada focuses on vibrations and radiations of life energy using sound. Like other therapies that use bells, drums, and musical recordings to enhance health and healing processes, this yoga may affect the body via the endocrine system.

❑ Kundalini seems to awaken the primal force (*kundalini*), which sleeps like a coiled snake at the base of the spine, through contemplation and/or Tantra, a sexual way to raise kundalini—but don't get excited: *celibacy* and turning one's sexual energy to God is Tantra's ultimate goal.

❑ Hatha also seeks integration of different aspects of self to attain a relaxed health and harmony of mind and body. Identified with the sun (*Ha*) and moon (*Tha*), it is sometimes called the gentle yoga. Breathing routines and *asanas* focus on mastery over the body and the *chakras*, or energy centers, in the body.

Several twentieth-century versions of the above, traditional yogas from the *Yoga Sutras,* have been and are being developed by modern gurus, teachers, and their students.

❑ Integral yoga was first developed by the modern guru Sri Aurobindo. It is a synthesis of traditional yogas and their goals with a warning "against extreme tendencies which mislead people into lopsided development." For example, hatha yoga may seduce its students into pursuing physical feats at the expense of higher spiritual values and activities. Integral yoga's ultimate aim is self-integration, including love, knowledge, wisdom, action, and peace. Swami Satchidananda also calls his school of yoga "Integral Yoga." The name seems to show the intention of creating a yoga of the whole being.

❑ Iyengar-style Hatha, developed by B.S.K. Iyengar and his students, is an example of a modern adaptation of Hatha yoga. Iyengar teaches Jumpings, or brisk Sun Salutations (usually a meditative flowing of several asanas together to greet the sunrise). Done long and hard enough, Jumpings can raise the heart rate into the aerobic training zone for a cardiovascular workout. Another, low-impact aerobic workout designed by Mary Pullig Schatz, M.D. is a series of flowing, standing poses.

Hatha yoga, especially Iyengar-style Hatha yoga, and Integral Yoga are the most widely available of the more physically-oriented versions.

Doing Yoga

Yoga exercises are used primarily to build and maintain a healthy mind, body, and spirit. The practices are much more than just the positions and breathing emphasized by the more physically-oriented branches. Cleansing routines and diet restriction, closely allied with yoga's mother culture's medical system, Ayurveda, are also recommended. Yogic philosophy and psychology includes moral and mental training. The goal of *samadhi,* to realize our perfect union with the Universal Force or God, requires mastery over all parts of one's life and being.

When looking for a teacher or a class to start learning yoga, ask what kind of yoga is taught, how active it is, and what kind of cool-down or meditation is included. Some teachers and their styles are more strenuous than others. Hatha yoga, a more gentle and breath-oriented style, is the best known and most popular. Remember Richard Hittleman on your local PBS station back in the '60s and '70s? Today you can catch other yoga instructors in those very early or late time slots.

Yoga has also been adapted for the elderly. *Easy Does It Yoga* is a "self-help program for total physical and mental fitness for older people." It includes special exercises to do in bed, a wheelchair, or the tub!

Most of my friends who practice yoga do it with the discipline of a devotee, practicing every day. I can see the benefits in their physical health as well as mental attitudes. I have made several attempts to get into the good habit of yoga, including a week-long retreat in the Big Sur mountains learning Iyengar-style yoga. The difference between Hatha and Iyengar-inspired yoga, in my experience, is the difference between Mr. Rogers and Clint Eastwood. Choose your style!

I'm afraid that my yogic discipline has fallen into a rather limited practice of a few stretches to jump-start the old body first thing in the morning. I have also used Acu-Yoga positions during my candida healing program. It helped with allergic headaches and sluggish intestines.

Applications and Cautions

While the extraordinary physical feats performed by Indian yogis are impressive, yogic techniques and principles include applications for us common folk. Doctors in England are using biofeedback and yoga to teach patients to lower and control blood pressure. B.S.K. Iyengar works with medical patients in Puna, India. He emphasizes yoga's "squeezing and soaking'" action on certain organs, such as the pancreas, to reduce a diabetic's need for insulin, or on the thyroid to stimulate an underactive gland.

Yoga has been integrated into holistic approaches to pain control. Various kinds of chronic pain have been reduced through a combined therapy program that included autogenic relaxation, diaphragmatic breathing, diet and nutrition counseling, biofeedback, meditation, psychotherapy, and Hatha yoga exercises.

Yoga is also used as an exercise for general conditioning of the body, especially in health recovery. Different yogas can be used for different benefits.

Beyond the general health conditioning benefits, specific poses are sometimes identified as affecting particular organs or physiological systems. Because any practice of yoga can produce physiological changes, individuals under treatment for a specific treatment should check with their primary care providers before that first class to see if yoga will help, not harm, the treatment program.

The yoga poses, if done incorrectly, for too long, or too strenuously, can cause physical damage, particularly to the back. One friend injuried his upper spine (cervical vertebrae) by holding the Plough asana too long. Training in the beginning and on-going classes, and supervision as you progress, are important to making yoga a healthy practice.

Most important, aerobic yoga requires all the cautions of doing aerobics: a complete cardivascular and structural evaluation to determine whether, how hard, and how long to exercise; stretching before and after the workout; and including warm-up, cool-down, and relaxation periods in the routine.

Finally, Dr. Motoyama and others point out that yoga, when pursued with discipline, can develop extrasensory, paranormal, or spiritual awareness. Yoga is designed as a holistic system; hopefully the meditative aspects, coupled with improved physical health, will prepare each student for whatever new perspective on self and life may arise.

READ MORE ABOUT IT

YOGA

Light On Yoga
by B.K.S. Iyengar
(New York: Schocken Books, 1966/1976)

Freedom from Stress: A Holistic Approach
by Phil Nuernberger, Ph.D.
(Honesdale, Pa: Himalayan International Institute, 1981)

Integral Yoga: The Concept of Harmonious and Creative Living
by Haridas Chaudhuri
(Wheaton, IL: Quest Books, 1974)

Yoga and Psychotherapy: The Evolution of Consciousness
by Swami Rama and Rudolph Ballentine, M.D.
(Honesdale, PA: Himalayan International Institute, 1976)

Yoga Psychology: A Practical Guide to Meditation
by Swami Ajaya, Ph.D.
(Honesdale, PA: Himalayan International Institute, 1976/1983)

Easy Does It Yoga for Older People
by Alice Christensen and David Rankin
(San Francisco: Harper & Row, 1979)

Runner's World Yoga Book
by Jean M. Couch
(Mountain View, CA: Runner's World Books, 1979)

RESOURCES

Yoga Journal (published by)
California Yoga Journal Association
2054 University Avenue
Berkeley, CA 94704
(415) 841-9200
❑ annual directory of teachers and centers
❑ annual directory of retreats
❑ membership
❑ networking
❑ publications

Iyengar Yoga Institute
2404 27th Avenue
San Francisco, CA 94116
(415) 753-0909
❑ information
❑ classes and trainings

Himalayan International Institute of Yoga, Science and Philosophy
RR1, Box 400
Honesdale, PA 18431
(717) 253-5551
❑ information
❑ retreats
❑ publications

Integral Yoga Institute
227 West 13th Street
New York, NY 10011
(212) 929-0586
❑ classes

Ananda Community
14618 Tyler Foote Road
Nevada City, CA 95959
(916) 292-3494
❑ information
❑ classes
❑ training
❑ publications
❑ products
❑ speakers

A Last Word
or Two

◇ **T**he title for this book, *Encyclopedia,* signals an intention to be all-inclusive. In the early days of the holistic health movement, that might have been possible. There were only so many pioneering practitioners rediscovering or inventing new ways to treat body, mind, and spirit. Also, many of the "alternative" medicines were sequestered in the "new age" reserves like Esalen, Findhorn, and other pockets of enlightenment scattered around the world.

Today, resource directories available in many cities, like the San Francisco Bay Area's *Commonground,* list hundreds of practitioners of healing arts and many different therapies. My mother sends me clippings from conservative Midwestern newspapers like the *Chicago Tribune* on everything from massage therapy to past life regression. The new health awareness is everywhere.

The Encyclopedia of Alternative Health Care is about the classics, the basics, those healing arts most available to the new health care consumer. The "Healing Arts" section profiles most of the major new directions in lifestyle health and complementary medicines. This is only the beginning.

While I name a number of variations and related healing arts in chapters about original developments, I know I have not covered everything that is out there. It is in the nature of human beings and the health care industry to continually change, grow, and evolve.

New therapies, especially new composite systems, are ripening into practical healing modalities at this moment. Ancient knowledge and ideas that were discounted in the rush toward a rational and scientific world are reemerging. They are being rediscovered, and refined, explored for these times, developed by the new pioneers, scientists, and investigators.

The settler generation of practitioners, those who have followed the early pioneers, are evolving their own styles within each established modality. Some healers combine many different arts, creating original approaches to healing, treatment of chronic complaints, and establishing a healthy lifestyle. Practitioners today are devising the Polarities, Applied Kinesiology, or Bioenergetics of tomorrow.

They are doing it by learning from their clients—from how their clients heal and grow. Your experiences and your feedback about them are part of the creative process. Clients contribute to the direction and refinement of the new health care as much as do doctors, scientists, researchers, practitioners, and healers. We *are* the new health awareness because we are living it today.

I want to hear about your experiences, your new awareness, and what is developing in the new health fields today. If, on your own journey toward better health, you discover a terrific new practitioner or healing modality that you would like to share with me, write to me.

Tell me what you have discovered: how it works and/or how it has worked for you. What effect has it had on your health and your life? Why? Or, if you had a "bad" experience, what happened and why? What might have been the problem?

You are the new health care consumers. You vote or create the market with your dollars, your feedback, your word-of-mouth on who and what is good or bad. More and more of you are taking charge of your bodies, choosing what may become major new tools for a healthy lifestyle by choosing whether or not to use complementary healing arts.

I want to know what you have found or learned, whether you have found a great practitioner or a terrific new healing art, and what you are thinking and experiencing.

Please write me at:

Kristin Gottschalk Olsen
c/o Pocket Books
1230 Avenue of the Americas
New York, NY 10020

Bibliography

(Other books are listed in individual chapters' reading lists)

Aihara, Herman. *Acid and Alkaline*. Oroville, CA: George Ohsawa Macrobiotic Foundation, 1971/1986.

Ardell, Donald B. *High Level Wellness: An Alternative to Doctors, Drugs, and Disease*. New York: Bantam Books, 1977/1979.

Ausubel, Ken. "The Troubling Case of Harry Hoxley." *New Age Journal*, Vol. V, No. 4 (July/August): 42–49.

Bliss, Shepard, ed. *The New Holistic Health Handbook: Living Well in the New Age*. Lexington, MA: Stephen Greene Press, 1985.

Berkeley Holistic Health Center, comp. *The Holistic Health Life Book: A Guide to Personal and Planetary Well-Being*. Berkeley, CA: And/Or Press, 1981

_____*The Holistic Health Handbook*. Berkeley, CA: And/Or Press, 1978.

Blair, Lawrence. *Rhythms of Vision: the Changing Patterns of Belief*. New York: Schocken Books, 1976.

Consumers Union, ed. *Health Quackery*. Mt. Vernon, NY: Consumers Union, 1980.

Coulter, Harris Livermore. *Divided Legacy: A History of the Schism in Medical Thought*, Vols. 1–3. Washington, D.C.: Weehawken, 1975.

Duffy, John. *The Healers: A History of American Medicine*. Urbana, IL: University of Illinois Press, 1979.

Dunn, Terence. "The Practice and Spirit of T'ai Chi Ch'uan." *Yoga Journal* 77 (November/December 1987): 62–65.

Ferguson, Tom. *Medical Self-Care: Access to Health Tools*. New York: Summit Books, 1980.

Fletcher, Sally. *The Challenge of Epilepsy*. Santa Rosa: Aura Publishing, 1985.

Flynn, Patricia Anne Randolph. *Holistic Health: The Art and Science of Care*. Bowie, Maryland: Robert J. Brady, 1980.

Frager, Robert and James Fadiman. *Personality and Personal Growth*. New York: Harper and Row, 1984.

Friedman, Milton. "From Poland with Prana." *New Realities* Vol. VII, No. 6 (July/August 1987): 10–15.

323

Geis, Larry and Alta Picchi Kelly, ed. *The New Healers: Healing the Whole Person*. Berkeley, CA: And/Or Press, 1980.

Grossinger, Richard. *Planet Medicine: From Stone Age Shamanism to Post-Industrial Healing*. Boulder, Co: Shambhala, 1982.

Hastings, Arthur C., James Fadiman, and James S. Gordon, ed. *Health for the Whole Person: Complete Guide to Holistic Medicine*. Toronto: Bantam Books, 1981.

Heller, Joseph and William A. Henkin. *Bodywise*. Los Angeles: Jeremy P. Tarcher, 1986.

Higgins, Melissa. "Mary Burmeister, Master of Jin Shin Jyutsu." *Yoga Journal* 79 (March/April 1988): 24–29.

Hutchinson, Michael. "Exploring the Inner Sea." *New Age Journal* (May 1984): 21–26.

Kaptchuk, Ted and Michael Croucher. *The Healing Arts: Exploring the Medical Ways of the World*. New York: Summit Books, 1987.

Keleman, Stanley. *Emotional Anatomy: the Structure of Experience*. Berkeley, CA: Center Press, 1985.

Kogan, Gerald. *Your Body Works: A Guide to Health, Energy, and Balance*. Berkeley, CA: And/Or Press, 1980.

Kruger, Helen. *Other Healers, Other Cures*. Indianapolis, IN: Bobbs-Merrill Co., 1974.

LeShan, Lawrence. *The Mechanic and the Gardener: Making the Most of the Holistic Revolution in Medicine*. New York: Holt, Rinehart and Winston, 1982.

Leviton, Richard. "Moving with Milton Trager." *East West: The Journal of Natural Health and Living*, Vol. 18, No. 1 (January 1988): 55–60.

Low, Jeffrey. "The Modern Body Therapies: A First Hand Look at Leading Bodywork Therapies." *Massage Magazine*, Issue 13 (April/May 1988): 48–50.

Lucus, Richard. *Nature's Medicine: The Folklore, Romance and Value of Herbal Remedies*. North Hollywood, CA: Wilshire Books, 1969.

Mann, A.T. *The Round Art: The Astrology of Time and Space*. New York: W. H. Smith Publishers, 1979.

Mattson, Phyllis H. *Holistic Health in Perspective*. Palo Alto: Mayfield Publishing, 1982.

Olsen, Kristin Gottschalk. "Managing Your Health: On Becoming a Participating Health Client." Master's thesis, John F. Kennedy University, 1987.

Podolsky, Doug M. and Cathy Sears. "Ayurveda: Pulse Reading, Herbs and Oil Massage." *American Health Magazine* (July/August 1988): 78–81.

Quinn, Janet. "Therapeutic Touch: The Empowerment of Love." *New Realities* Vol. VII, No. 5 (May/June 1987): 21–26.

Salmon, J. Warren, ed. *Alternative Medicines: Popular and Policy Perspectives*. New York: Travistock Publications, 1984.

Samuels, Mike and Hal Bennett. *The Well Body Book*. New York, Random House, 1973.

Schwartz, Gary E. and Jackson Beatty. *Biofeedback: Theory and Research*. New York: Academic Press, 1977.

Simply Living. "Increase Your Life Span Through Ayurvedic Medicine" by Dr. Deepak Chopra. Vol. 3, No. 3, 1988, p. 26–29.

Singer, Charles and E. Ashworth Underwood. *A Short History of Medicine*. New York: Oxford University Press, 1962.

Stanway, Andrew. *Alternative Medicine: A Guide to Natural Therapies*. London: Rainbird Publishing Group, 1979.

Starhawk. *The Spiral Dance: A Rebirth of the Ancient Religion of the Great Goddess*. San Francisco: Harper & Row, 1979.

Steiger, Brad. "Taking On the Medical Establishment: An Arizona Homeopath Fights Back and Wins." *East West: The Journal of Natural Health and Living*, Vol. 17, No. 5 (May 1987): 73–76.

Ullman, Dana. "Royal Medicine." *New Age Journal* Vol. III, No. 5 (September/October 1987): 45–52.

Weil, Andrew. *Health and Healing*. Boston: Houghton, Mifflin, 1988.

Weiss, Kay, ed. *Women's Health Care: A Guide to Alternatives*. Reston, VA: Reston Publishing, 1984.